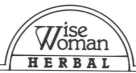

HERBAL
FOR THE CHILDBEARING YEAR

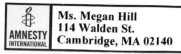
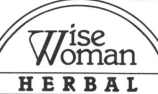

Wise Woman HERBAL

FOR THE CHILDBEARING YEAR

Susun S. Weed

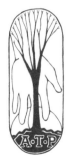

Ash Tree Publishing
Woodstock, New York

All information in this *Wise Woman Herbal* is based on the experiences and research of the author and other professional healers. This information is shared with the understanding that you accept complete responsibility for your own health and well-being. You have a unique body and the action of each herbal medicine is unique and health care is full of variables. The results of any treatment suggested herein cannot always be anticipated and never guaranteed. The author and publisher are not responsible for any adverse effects or consequences resulting from the use of any remedies, procedures, or preparations included in this *Wise Woman Herbal*. Consult your inner guidance, knowledgeable friends, and trained healers in addition to the words written here.

May the six directions empower this medicine work.
May it be pleasing to my grandmothers, the ancient ones.
And may it be of benefit to all beings.

So mote it be.

Contents

Acknowledgements

I think it's obvious; a book is made by a group of people, not one individual. I asked the people who joined me in creating and producing this book to help me fill it with love, joy, and cooperation. And they did. I especially want to thank:

- Clove, for editing and proofing all the versions, and counseling and supporting me through the entire process.
- Pauline Oliveros, for providing technical support, including the use of her Apple II plus and Wordstar software, and access to her copy maker.
- Anne Frye, Valerie Hobbs, Jennifer Houston, Dev Kirn Khalsa, and BJ Miller, for reading and correcting my information, for sharing their wisdom and experiences, and for encouraging and teaching me.
- Janice Novet, for her spirit-filled illustrations; and Janet Woodman, for creating my vision of a perfect cover.
- Peter Blum, for typesetting endlessly; Peggy Goddard, for pasting-up perfectly; and Barry Koffler and Clove, for indexing thoroughly.
- Cynthia Werthamer, for early editing and structural advice.
- And all the Wise Women midwives, who must remain nameless to protect themselves, for nurturing me, and for insisting that this book be born.

Green blessings to all!

Foreword

Women are carriers of life. We hold the fruit of our loving beneath our hearts. For too long we have lost touch with the fullness of this mystery due to modern, technological culture.

Wise Woman Herbal is another ally in reclaiming our lost gnosis as healers for ourselves and one another. It demonstrates beyond doubt that now is the time to be fully who we are throughout the childbearing year—guardians and nurturers of new life.

Susun S. Weed has created a magnificent testimony that the wise woman within is irrepressible. SHE will arise in all her glory if we but open our souls to our natural world. True to the essence of the herbs themselves, the material is presented mythically, botanically and lovingly. Susun not only introduces the novice to plant allies but further refines the already practicing herbalist's relationship with healing the fertility cycle.

It is challenging to choose one particular part as outstanding, as I found it all to be consistently excellent. Even after many years teaching herbal workshops to perinatal professional and natural parents, and mothering five children myself, I found much new and helpful material. It is kindred to my work—just like the book I would like to write.

In the many years since I wrote *Hygieia: A Woman's Herbal,* I have re-visioned my personal relationship with herbs to exclude their usage for abortions. I cannot endorse emmenagogic prescription in cases of pregnancy no matter how new the embryo. As a healer I strive to be harmless. With this clarification I heartily endorse Susun's wonderful book, for within its pages is distilled much worthwhile wisdom for mothers and mothers-to-be. This book is sweet word-medicine.

Wise Woman Herbal is a book I would give my best friend— and her daughter contemplating pregnancy. I will certainly share it with my sister-midwives. It speaks to the deepest needs of women wishing their childbearing year (and years) to be the best that it can.

Blessed Be Gentle Mother!

With Love,
Jeannine Parvati Baker,
Utah 1985

P.S. Here's a terrific miscarriage preventative formula used by the Utah midwives with great success. I gave it to one pregnant woman with a chronic "incompetent" cervix who had lost 5 babies and delivered all her others early. She began miscarriage once again, faithfully took this formula, and carried full term! A miracle, everyone called it. The formula is one ounce Wild Yam, one ounce Squaw Vine, one ounce False Unicorn root, one half ounce Cramp Bark. Simmer for 20 minutes in one quart water. Take one wineglassful every four hours until symptoms of miscarriage cease. They will!

Introduction

The childbearing year is a thirteen month year: the two months before conception, the nine months of pregnancy, and the two months following the birth. The childbearing year is a time of change and an opportunity to grow, filled with rapid physical adjustments and fierce emotions. The childbearing year touches every season. This book is about herbs for the childbearing year.

For more than a million years Wise Women have used herbs—gathered, eaten, tended, loved herbs—and taught their daughters the wisdom of herbs in the childbearing year.

In Europe, five hundred years ago, men tortured and burned the Wise Women who healed with herbs, the midwives, the ones who celebrated the cyclical ways. Calling them witches, they burned them in millions and broke the flow of mother to daughter transmission. In the Americas, their sons down the way killed the medicine women and curanderas, the Wise Women of the New World. Then they denied the existence of Wise Women in history.

Without our connections to each other and the earth, without our mothers' wisdom, we forgot our power. When we were told that we had no souls, and no minds, and no sisters, we believed it was true. When they told us that childbearing was too dangerous and difficult for women, midwives, and herbs, we believed it was true.

But the Wise Women live in our dreams, our visions, our deepest memories. We hear their whispers and we listen.

Wise Woman healing works in cycles and seasons, with the turning of the planets, and the pulsation of life. Wise Women gather each herb at its time and use it to nourish and build the sixty million cells we each create every second. They understand the attunement built into our cells after thousands of generations nourished on wild foods, the special kinship our bodies have with the vital elements condensed in herbs.

Wise Women herbalists see the whole herb, the physical forces and the subtle forces, and respect this wholeness. Wise Women make use of the color, form, spirit, and substance of a plant, using it as a whole, not dividing it into parts and seeing power only in the "active" principle. Wise Women know that we are each whole and unique, in an individual, everchanging, symbiotic relationship with herbs.

Wise Woman healing is grounded, earthed, rooted. The Wise Woman accepts herself and her changes, her moods and her bleedings. She tends to birthing and dying without alienation from herself or the ones she helps. She is open to the life song surrounding her, she hears the secrets of the herbs. Fairies appear to her; devas bless her. All that she needs for health and well being grows within the fall of her foot. She prepares the nourishment, she concocts the medicines. She is filled with creativity. Her life, her children, her art, her healing are shaped by her understanding of color, tone, harmony, and balance. She is wise in the ways of heart, body, and spirit.

This book speaks to the Wise Woman in you—the pregnant woman—and to the Wise Woman in your mate, lover, midwife, doctor, childbirth educator, and friends. It is based on the belief that you are capable of observing your own body, heart, and mind, responding to the messages you receive during the childbearing year, and caring for yourself in a context of loving support and assistance.

The information I share with you here represents the careful experiments and experiences of many herbalists and ordinary people. It is not a compendium of herbal remedies gathered from other books with the hope that these herbs will work, but a record of herbal practices which have been tested in many situations and with a wide variety of people. I see this work as a link in remembering ourselves as Wise Women, joining with the Wise Women in China and other areas where herbal medicine has an unbroken tradition, joining with the Wise Women in plants, joining with the Wise Woman mothering earth.

Do you remember? Is that a picture of your grandmother in her garden? We are all Wise Women.

Using This Book

• Start by looking through the whole book quickly one time. Childbearing is not neatly divided into chapters. Remedies are discussed when the problem arises, but may be best used before the problem occurs. For example: remedies for breech presentation are much more effective if used well before the onset of labor, when the presentation becomes a problem.

• Pay particular attention to Chapter Six, Herbal Pharmacy. Best results and safety are dependent on your ability to use the correct amount of herb and the correct preparation. Don't assume you already know how to make the herbal medicines mentioned, even if you've been working with herbs for years. For example: I suggest infusions throughout this book, using one ounce of dried herb in two to four cups of water and steeping for up to eight hours; an infusion is not a cup of tea.

• Then look up your particular area of interest or problem. Try a mild remedy first. Wise Woman healing proceeds in this order (when life is not threatened): 1) Do nothing; the body heals itself. 2) Use a homeopathic remedy or flower essence; the vibration of a plant is harmless but healing. 3) Use herbs and foods, especially wild greens, to nourish and tone the body or a particular organ; billions of your cells are replaced each minute. 4) Cautiously take cleansing or potentially toxic herbs; side effects are more likely when alkaloid-rich plants are consumed. 5) Use concentrated, refined, or synthesized herbal medicines; these are commonly known as drugs. 6) Intervene with surgery; healing is complicated and likelihood of infection is increased when surgery is used. **It is my experience that herbal medicines do not interfere with, nullify, or potentize chemical medicines unless they are taken at the same time.** It is, for instance, safe to use Blue Cohosh or labor tincture to augment contractions, and follow this, after 20-30 minutes, with Pitocin, if necessary.

• Use herbs preventatively. Preventative medicine is one of the foundations of the Wise Woman tradition. Remedies for some postpartum problems, used during labor, prevent the problem. Remedies for newborn jaundice, taken during pregnancy, prevent the occurrence of jaundice. And so on.

• To ensure safety, check the index for the Latin name of the plant remedy you intend to use. Identify all plants, even if you buy them in a store or by mail, with their Latin names. The Latin binomial is specific to one plant; common names vary and overlap. For example: Boneset may refer to *Symphytum officinale* or to *Eupatorium perfoliatum.*

• Use the index to help you find more information on an herb you are using. Wise Woman teaching is based on cycles, so instead of centralizing all the information on each plant, I have cycled it throughout the book. If we took a walk together, we'd encounter the same plant several times, learning something new and different and restating previous information each time. That's how this book works, too.

• Look up *italicized words* in the glossary.

• Make use of the references and resources at the end of each chapter.

★ My favorite remedies, or herbs which are used successfully by a majority of midwives and mothers, are starred.

• Add your own marginal notes. I've written in some comments and lots of common herb names to start you off. Make note of remedies you use and the results you experience, etc.

• Trust your sense of what's right for you. Use this book in conjunction with your own inner Wise Woman. Seek second and third opinions. You are unique. Respect your body, your intuitions, and your feelings.

• Enjoy!

Using Herbs Safely

As the accessibility of herbal medicines has grown over the past twenty years (after an enforced decline spanning many decades), questions of safety have also grown. Scare stories abound of carcinogens found in herbs, poisonous plants mistakenly sold as curative ones, and allergic reactions to supposedly safe herbs. When you begin to use herbs as part of your health program, you may wonder how to use them safely. To avoid complexity, risk, and unneeded worry: .

• Begin by using gentle nourishing and tonic herbs; avoid plants that may be toxic.
• Use one herb at a time.
• Learn about one wild plant at a time from an experienced guide.
• Seek out the miracle medicines on your own doorstep.
• Remember that crude herbs (as opposed to the refined extracts known as drugs) rarely cause fatal allergic reactions or severely disabling side effects.
• Realize that reports of herbs having cancer-causing properties are misleading. They are usually based on studies done with purified extracts rather than whole plants. Alfalfa, Comfrey, Coltsfoot, and Sassafras each have a component that may be carcinogenic or mutagenic. When the "active" components are extracted and "purified," they may injure or mutate cells. But there are no reported cases of cancer from the thousands of people who have used these herbs for well-being and health care through the centuries, for these "active" components are only a tiny fraction of the plant material, and the large amount of "passive" components buffers and neutralizes them.
• Build up a foundation of trust in the healing effectiveness of plants by using remedies for minor problems and first aid before you try to deal with serious health problems.
• Increase your herbal knowledge through direct experience, experimentation, and reading.

• Gather a support group of people interested in "alternative" medicines and consult them when you feel unsure.

• Respect the power of plants; those strong enough to act as medicines affect the body and spirit in powerful ways.

• Respect the strength of herbs; some plants are so potent that they can only be used in minute quantities.

• Respect the unique individuality of every plant, every person, and every situation.

• Understand the varying effects and side effects of nourishing, tonic, cleansing, and potentially toxic plants.

Nourishing herbs are the safest of all herbs; they rarely have any side effects. Nourishing herbs may generally be taken in any quantity and for extended periods of time. They act in the body as food, providing nutrients such as vitamins, minerals, proteins, simple sugars, and starches. They improve existing conditions by strengthening the body's defenses and resources. Nourishing herbs used in this *Wise Woman Herbal* include: Alfalfa, barley, Borage, Comfrey, Nettles, Parsley, Raspberry leaf, Red Clover, and Slippery Elm.

Tonic herbs act slowly in the body and have a cumulative effect; they are most beneficial when used consistently for months. Tonics rarely give rise to side effects. They generally aid the body to balance its energy and function more easily and dependably. Some tonic herbs are bitter; this taste is an indication that these herbs should be taken in small amounts. Other tonic herbs have a bland or soothing taste and can be taken safely in large amounts. Tonic herbs used in this *Wise Woman Herbal* include: Blessed Thistle, Burdock, Dandelion, Liferoot, Sarsaparilla, Skullcap, and Yellow Dock.

Cleansing herbs stimulate the body's cleansing systems and disease fighting mechanisms. They are also called antibiotics, antiseptics, and antibacterials. Cleansing herbs are very strong in their effects and are more likely to have side effects. They are usually taken in small amounts for short periods of time. They may stress some parts of the body in order to help other parts, or may be too powerful in their effect for some people. Use with care. Cleansing herbs used in this *Wise Woman Herbal* include: Echinacea, Elder root, Golden Seal, Rosemary, Sage, Uva Ursi, and Yarrow.

Potentially toxic or "poisonous" **herbs** are the most potent medicines of all. They stimulate powerful healing and releasing actions in the body. An overdose will almost always cause side effects. Potentially toxic herbs are taken for a short period of time or in very small doses. Potentially toxic herbs used in this *Wise Woman Herbal* include: Pennyroyal, Poke, Black Cohosh, Blue

Cohosh, Cayenne, Cotton, Dong Quai, Licorice, Lobelia, Mistletoe, and Tansy. Increase your herbal knowledge and sense of security when using these potentially toxic herbs by consulting other herbal references. It is especially important to check further on the possible side effects of any of the potentially toxic herbs if you are allergic to foods or medicines.

The herbs gathered here in the *Wise Woman Herbal for the Childbearing Year* are accessible and safe. By accessible, I mean that they are easily found growing nearby you, or that you can readily buy them at health food stores, herbal apothecaries, or through the mail. By safe, I mean that they will not cause harm, now or later, if used with respect and knowledge.

The most important thing to remember is that the body heals itself, and you can assist and strengthen that healing process with wise use of herbs.

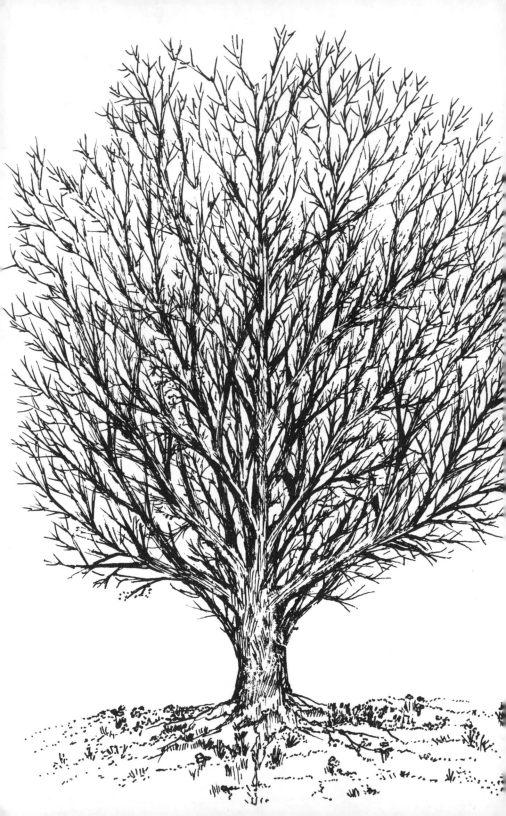

Before Pregnancy

Before pregnancy is fertility. Desiring pregnancy, you desire fertility. Avoiding pregnancy, you perceive fertility as a problem.

Information on herbs which affect fertility—beneficially or adversely—is scarce and often dangerously vague when available. A look through my well-stocked library of modern herbals reveals very little about herbal fertility control. The World Health Organization began compiling a computer data base of plants used for controlling conception in the late seventies, but their results are not generally available. Herbs used before pregnancy are mentioned in older herbals and in anthropological accounts of aboriginal peoples. But these references (and current herbals which repeat from them) tend to be very general, hardly ever specifying an exact dosage or potential side effects. Our foremothers knew how to use herbs to promote or prevent pregnancy, but much of their wisdom is lost or destroyed.

What can be done to fill this void? I share with you my own experiences, feedback from my students, Wise Woman memories, and information gleaned from a wide range of published and unpublished resources. From the hundreds of herbs and substances reputed to influence fertility, I have picked remedies for you that have shown themselves to be effective and safe when used with caution and respect. Although it is my experience that these herbs will not cause harm, I ask you to remember that herbs do not always have predictable effects. The same plant may increase fertility in one person and decrease it in another. Differences in preparation may change temporary birth control to permanent sterility. The effective substances in some plants may be present only at certain times of the year.

If you hope to conceive soon or wish to prevent pregnancy, consider the herbs and the green *devas* who stand ready to help you.

Fertility Promoters

The reasons for infertility are complex and differ greatly from woman to woman and couple to couple. Despite these complexities, I have found that it is often amazingly easy and straightforward to establish a pregnancy with the help of herbs.

Herbs used to encourage a pregnancy are characterized by their ability to 1) nourish and tonify the uterus, 2) nourish the entire body, 3) relax the nervous system, 4) establish and balance normal functioning of the hormonal system, and 5) balance sexual desire.

Causes of infertility:
50% = weak sperm
35% = blocked tubes
15% = unknown

★ **Red Clover flowers**   The single most useful herb for establishing fertility is *Trifolium pratense.* Its high vitamin content is especially useful for the uterus; its high protein content aids the entire body; its profuse and exceedingly absorbable calcium and magnesium relax the nervous system and promote fertility; its high mineral content, including virtually every trace mineral needed by the glands, helps restore and balance hormonal functions. In addition, Red Clover alkalinizes the body and may balance the acid/alkaline level of the vagina and uterus in favor of conception.

Red Clover is in the pea/bean family. Add fresh flowers to salad. Cook a handful of dried flowers in with your rice.

Red Clover is often combined with Peppermint in fertility brews since Mints are safe and pleasant tasting sexual stimulants. Infuse one ounce of Red Clover blossoms and a teaspoon of Peppermint (or any other Mint) in a quart of water for four hours. This infusion may be taken freely throughout the day and for several months continuously. Alfalfa is regarded as a substitute for Red Clover, but I do not find it as effective.

• **Nettle leaves**   The common stinging Nettle, *Urtica dioica,* is a uterine tonic and general nourisher with a special ability to strengthen the kidneys and adrenals. Its high mineral and chlorophyll content makes it an excellent food and tonic for the hormonal system. These characteristics make Nettle infusion my second favorite brew for increasing fertility. As with Red Clover, drink one or more cups of the infusion daily for several months.

● Red Raspberry leaves   All *Rubus* species, but most especially the wild ones, provide leaves which contain an effective uterine tonic and a large amount of calcium. Raspberry leaf is my third choice as an herbal fertility promoter. It is most effective when combined with Red Clover. One or more cups of the infusion (prepared by steeping one half ounce Red Clover blossoms and one half ounce Raspberry leaves in a quart of water for four hours) can be taken daily and continued for months. Another way to increase the fertility promoting ability of Raspberry is to add 5-15 drops of either Dong Quai root tincture or False Unicorn root tincture to each cup of Raspberry leaf infusion.

● Dong Quai root   I have found *Angelica sinensis* invaluable in normalizing menstrual periods. It is widely and highly regarded as a fertility promoter. The form I favor is a water-based combination extract sold in Chinatown stores under the name "Tang Kwei Gin." Best results are obtained when Dong Quai preparations are taken during the days between ovulation and menstruation and discontinued from the beginning of the menstrual flow to ovulation. If the "Gin" is unavailable, substitute a homemade Dong Quai/Comfrey root tincture. (See Appendix II.)   CAUTION: Use Dong Quai only in combination with other herbs.

● False Unicorn root   *Chamaelirium luteum* is regarded as a powerful and positive uterine tonic. It is also believed to have a strong beneficial and alkalinizing influence on the ovaries, kidneys, and bladder. Always noted as "the" herb for infertility, False Unicorn root is difficult to obtain except in commercial combination tinctures and capsules. Dosage of the tincture is 5-15 drops per day. The infusion is taken in sips, up to half a cup daily.

● Ovulation is controlled by light. Leave a light on in your bedroom for three nights midway through your menstrual cycle; all other nights keep the room in total darkness. You will ovulate when the light is on. Have intercourse during the three "light" nights if you want to conceive. This method, called **lunaception,** combines well with herbs which promote fertility.

• Carlton Fredricks reports low levels of para-aminobenzoic acid (**PABA**) in women who have difficulty in conceiving, and increased success in conception with supplements of PABA, but does not give dosage information.

• **Calcium** and **magnesium** are the two minerals thought to be the most important in affecting a woman's ability to conceive and maintain a pregnancy. Refer to Appendix I for herbal sources of these minerals.

• There is a well-established link between vitamin E and fertility. **Vitamin E** is said to have a "dramatic" effect on the reproductive systems of both men and women. Five hundred to 1500 IU taken daily by the male partner for several months prior to conception has been shown to prevent birth defects in children of couples who had defective children. Wheat germ oil is my favorite natural source of vitamin E. For other sources, see Appendix I.

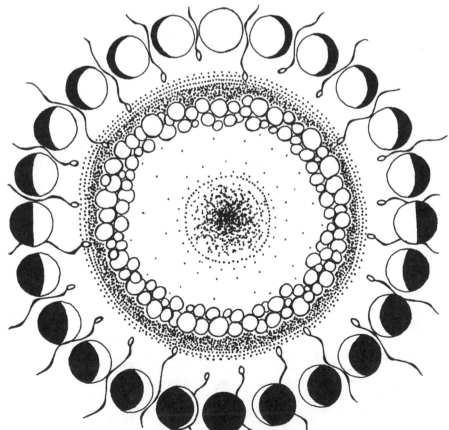

Herbal Birth Control

Herbal birth control is most effective when combined with knowledge of your fertility cycles, selective abstinence, mental control, and barriers to sperm. You may choose herbs to cause temporary or permanent sterility, to prevent implantation of a fertilized egg, to bring on a late menstrual flow, or to empty the uterus if you believe that conception has taken place. Although some of these herbs have potentially dangerous side effects, they are generally considered safe to use. Please respect their power.

Sterility Promoters

● **Stoneseed root**   *Lithospermum ruderale* was used by Shoshone women to cause permanent sterility. They prepared the root as a cold infusion, steeping it for several hours in cold, rather than boiling, water, and drank a cup daily for six months. Women of the Dakota tribes drank a root infusion or breathed the smoke from the burning plant to induce sterility. Another Stoneseed, the closely related *Lithospermum officinale*, is an old remedy for kidney failure due to blockage from stones.

● **Jack-in-the-Pulpit root**   *Arisaema triphyllum* was prepared by stirring one teaspoon of the dried, powdered root into a half cup of cold water. The strained liquid was drunk by Hopi women and supposedly prevented conception for one week. If permanent sterility was desired, two teaspoonsful were stirred into a cup of hot water and drunk. The eastern variety of this plant, *Arisaema atrorubens*, is thoroughly dried (some sources recommend for a full year) and then used as a foodstuff. CAUTION: The raw roots, actually corms, of *Arisaema* species contain calcium oxalate, which causes intense burning sensations in the mouth.

● **Thistles**   (*Carduus benedictus, Cnicus ochroncentrus* and some of the *Cirsiums*) Many types of Thistle seem to be useful in inhibiting fertilization. The Quinault

Indians used Thistles to induce temporary sterility by preparing an infusion of the entire plant in boiling water and drinking the resulting strong, bitter liquid. All varieties of Thistle are edible and I have enjoyed many meals of them, eating both the roots and the inner portion of the stem.

Artichokes are unopened Thistle buds.

Implantation Preventers

Herbs which prevent the implantation of a fertilized egg do so safely and relatively painlessly by making the *endometrium* unsuitable for the growth of the embryo. They are taken before or after the unprotected fertilizing intercourse. Positive results are indicated by a normal menstrual flow at the normal time. Women say that when they have used these herbs their flow has been somewhat heavier and has contained more clots than usual, circumstantial evidence of a pregnancy that didn't take. As there's been no controlled study of possible side effects from long and regular use of these herbs, they should not be used on a monthly basis. No known side effects accompany occasional use.

● **Wild Carrot seed**   One teaspoonful of the seeds of Queen Anne's Lace (*Daucus carota*) is taken daily, starting at the time of ovulation or immediately after unprotected intercourse during the fertile time, and continued for up to one week to prevent pregnancy. Women in Ragasthan, India use cultivated carrot seed in the same way. Researchers there have found that ingestion of carrot seed by mice prevents the implantation of their fertilized eggs. The seeds are oily and strong tasting, but not bitter or unpleasant. They are easily available for the taking in many areas of the world. Several species of Wild Carrot are abundant in all parts of North America, including city sidewalks, parks, and vacant lots. Wild Carrot seeds are not commercially available; if you plan on using cultivated carrot seeds, be absolutely certain they haven't been treated with toxic substances.

★ **Rutin**   Occurring naturally in association with vitamin C in many plant leaves, most notably Rue, buckwheat, and Elder, rutin can be used to prevent pregnancy. Take it as a tablet in doses of at least 500 mg daily for several days preceeding and following ovulation, or take it after fertilizing intercourse and continue until the menstrual flow begins.

● Smartweed leaves   *Polygonum hydropiper* grows as a weed all over the world and is used world-wide as a fertility regulator. It contains rutin, quercitin, and gallic acid, all of which interfere with normal pregnancy. Rutin inhibits the production of hormones which stimulate *gamete* production. Quercitin stimulates uterine contractions. Gallic acid is known as an anti-tumor agent; it may treat an embryo as a tumor and prevent its normal formation. Prepare an infusion of four ounces of the fresh or one ounce of the dried leaves in a quart of boiling water and drink freely until menstrual bleeding starts. Smartweed may be used to prevent implantation after intercourse during fertile days, or to bring on a missed period. It is almost certainly not safe to use unless you intend to follow up with a mechanical abortion should it not bring on the hoped-for discharge.

Menstrual Promoters

Herbs used to bring on or promote a menstrual flow are known as emmenagogues. There are at least fifty in common use throughout the world.

If your period is a day or two late, an emmenagogue may bring it on. If you suspect before your menstrual flow is due that you may be pregnant and wish not to be, begin drinking a menstrual promoter a week before your expected flow.

Some Good Emmenagogues

● Ginger root   Cultivated *Zingiber* is one of the strongest and fastest acting of the emmenagogues. I recall a friend dashing for the bathroom after drinking a Jamaican Ginger beer, saying: "But I'm not due to bleed until tomorrow!" The simplest way to prepare Ginger is to put one teaspoon of the powdered root into a cup and pour boiling water over it. Drink when it cools somewhat. Or make an infusion of one ounce of the whole dried root or the freshly grated root in a pint of water. Take no more than four cups a day of any of these brews. If you become nauseated by drinking Ginger, you have a strong

Spanish:
AJENJIBRE,
JENGIBRE

German:
INGWER

French:
GINGEMBRE

Chinese:
CHIANG

indication that you are pregnant. If your menstrual flow does not come within five days, discontinue use of Ginger.

● **Tansy leaves**   This prolific plant should not be confused with Tansy Ragwort, a potentially poisonous plant which is a weed in the midwest. The Tansy I am speaking of is *Tanacetum vulgare,* a garden plant or a wild plant of the northeast. It is a favorite of one of my students who has used it for years as a backup to her regular birth control. When necessary, she drinks an infusion of the flowers and leaves for a week before her period is due and claims that she has never been late yet. Other women have reported that they have used Tansy infusion successfully, but were disturbed by the temporary appearance of lumps in their breasts after use. There are also reports that Tansy can cause hemorrhage among women who normally have heavy menstrual flows. One midwife reports that she uses it as a tincture, giving 10 drops in a cup of warm water every two hours until bleeding begins. She says the tincture definitely induces abortion when the period is several weeks overdue.

● **Pennyroyal leaves**   The American variety of Pennyroyal, *Hedeoma pulegioides* is one of the most powerful of all emmenagogues. My first experience with using Pennyroyal as an abortifacient centered around a pregnant Great Dane. Her owner fasted her for three days, then fed her ground meat with several ounces of dried Pennyroyal mixed into it. She aborted one pup the next morning—but carried the other eight to term! They were all healthy and normal puppies. From this I have inferred that it is reasonably safe to try to abort with Pennyroyal, even if it doesn't work. But one midwife reports that in several instances women she knows have tried to abort (unsuccessfully) with Pennyroyal and their placentas have implanted dangerously low.

Pennyroyal is prepared as an infusion and taken as hot as possible; some women drink it in a hot bath. The tincture is taken in doses of 20 drops in a cup of hot water. No more than four cups of either preparation should be consumed per day and for no more than five days. This is considered sufficient to induce menstruation without taxing the woman. CAUTION: Half an ounce of Pennyroyal oil can cause death. **Do not use Pennyroyal oil internally.**

Also:
SQUAW MINT,
STINKING BALM,
THICKWEED,
FLEA CHASER

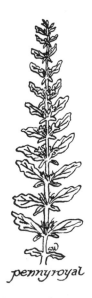

pennyroyal

★ Vitamin C   Ascorbic acid is the safest and reportedly most effective emmenagogue that can be used after the menstrual flow has failed to appear. Women report success even when three weeks "late." Six grams of vitamin C (6000 mg) is the daily dosage needed to abort. Take 500 mg every hour for 12 hours a day for up to six days. CAUTION: This dosage may produce loose stools.

A List of Emmenagogues

Don't exceed the recommended doses; many of these emmenagogues can cause strong side effects. The starred herbs (★) are *oxytocic;* use only with focused attention and acute sensitivity to the body's reactions. The herbs in **boldface** will bring on a late period about 60% of the time if the expected flow is no more than two weeks overdue.

• **Angelica** root: infusion, tincture (10 drops three times daily for four days)

• Fresh Lemon Balm leaves: tincture, bath

• Bethroot: infusion, tincture (a dropperful every four hours for five days)

★ Birthwort root or whole plant in flower: infusion

• Black Cohosh root: infusion, tincture (20 drops every six hours for four days)

★ Blue Cohosh root: infusion, tincture (20 drops every four hours for five days)

★ Cotton root bark: infusion

• European Vervain plant: tincture (15 drops every six hours for five days)

★ Ergot fungus: commercial extracts

• Feverfew plant in flower: tincture (40 drops every three hours for four days)

• Ginger root: infusion, tincture

• Hyssop leaves: infusion, tincture

• Liferoot plant in flower: tincture (20 drops twice daily for five days)

- Lovage root: infusion

★ Marijuana female flowers: infusion, tincture, smoke

★ Mistletoe leaves: infusion

- Motherwort plant: infusion

- Mugwort plant: decoction

- Osha root: infusion, tincture (10 drops every four hours for five days)

- **Fresh Parsley** leaves: juice, vaginal insert (several sprigs, changed twice daily for three days)

- **Pennyroyal** plant: infusion, tincture, oil (Avoid completely before and throughout pregnancy. Oil rubbed into skin may cause miscarriage.)

★ Peruvian bark: infusion, tincture (15 drops twice daily for four days)

- Rosemary plant in flower: infusion, tincture (20 drops twice daily for five days)

- **Rue** leaves: infusion, tincture (10 drops every six hours for four days)

- **Saffron** stigmas: one half gram daily for four days (ten grams is a fatal dose)

- Sumac berries: infusion (source of vitamin C and possibly rutin)

- Sweet Flag root: infusion, bath, tincture (10 drops every six hours for six days)

- **Tansy** plant in flower: infusion, tincture

- Fresh Wood Sorrel plant: infusion, tincture (10 drops every six hours for four days)

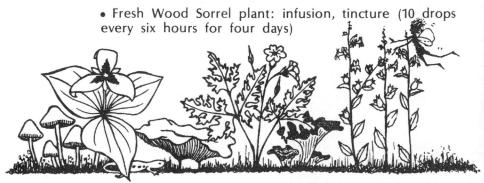

Uterine Contractors

Herbs which promote strong uterine contractions can cause an early miscarriage or abortion. Some uterine contractors are poisons, like Water Hemlock. Some herbs, such as certain seaweeds and pieces of Slippery Elm bark, are inserted into the os of the cervix to cause uterine contraction (and possible life threatening infection) by their irritating effect. Other herbs contain oxytocin, which encourages production of prostaglandins in the body; high levels of prostaglandins cause contraction of the uterus. A few herbs directly stimulate uterine contractions.

If your period is no more than two weeks late, you can probably abort by using a uterine contractor alone or in combination with a strong emmenagogue. Some women report success even when four weeks late. Abortion is a controversial subject, and herbal abortions are not an easy solution to the issues involved. Any abortion is physically, emotionally, and psychically stressful. If you decide that you are not going to nourish a life growing within, please seek a woman wise in the ways of bodies and feelings to help you.

● **Cotton root bark**   *Gossypium* is reported to be the safest and most certain herbal abortifacient. I have tried to obtain some organic Cotton root bark for six years now, without success. My information on its effectiveness comes from a study done by a women's health collective in New Mexico. They used an infusion taken by sips throughout the day until the abortion was well under way. This is apparently a traditional method of birth control among Native Americans who grow cotton. Specific information on dosage and possible side effects should be available to women who live in the South and seek out a traditional healer or *curandera*.

● **Blue Cohosh root**   *Caulophyllum thalictroides* is usually combined with Pennyroyal when used as an abortifacient. There are any number of ways to prepare and ingest this combination. Both Pennyroyal and Blue Cohosh are toxic in excess and can easily overtax the liver and kidneys. Headache and extreme nausea have been reported by many women using these herbs. This is a common remark: "I knew that if I could just drink one more cup of that infusion, I would abort, but I threw up every time I tried to!" CAUTION: Do not use Blue Cohosh if you have low blood pressure.

• Emmenagogue Formulae - See Appendix II

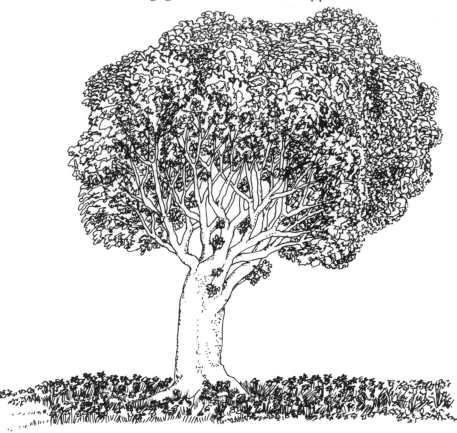

Teratogens

Substances that cause birth defects are known as teratogens. You and the fetus are particularly sensitive to teratogens during the first five months of the childbearing year (the two months prior to conception and the first three months of pregnancy). Exposure to teratogens interferes with the rhythmic reproductive dance of your genes, chromosomes, and cells. The effects of this disruption include infertility, miscarriage, low birth weight, and a wide range of mental and physical deformities in your baby. This list of teratogens is based on *Terata: A Mother's Prenatal Health Advisory* compiled by Jo Carrasco and Sue Keller. See References and Resources for reprint information.

Before and during pregnancy, completely avoid:

- Smoking

- Alcohol (including beer and wine)

- Raw or undercooked meat

- Radiation (x-rays, video display terminals)

- Caffeine (coffee, black tea, cola, chocolate, maté)

- DES (diethylstilbestrol)

- Aspirin

- Antihistamines, including *Ma-huang, Ephedra, Osha root*

- Most laxatives, including *Flax seed, Senna, Aloes, Castor Oil, Turkey Rhubarb, Buckthorn, Cascara Sagrada*

- Antacids

- Diuretics, including *Buchu, Horsetail, Juniper berries*

- pHisoHex (or anything else containing hexachlorophene)

- Hair dyes

- Hemorrhoid medications

- Chemical stimulants and depressants (LSD, psychotropics, phenobarbital, barbiturates, tranquilizers)

- Motion sickness or anti-nausea drugs (Bendectin)

- Epinephrine (Adrenalin) shots

- Sulfonamides (sulfa drugs) antibiotics

- Vaccines, anesthetics, mercury vapors in dentist's office

- Steroids and herbs containing steroid-like factors, including *Agave, Ginseng, Licorice, Hops, Sage* (which also decreases lactation)

- Hormones (birth control pills, most commercial meats)
- Acutane (acne medication)
- Excesses of vitamins A, C, or D (vitamins found naturally in herbs are safer than supplemental vitamin pills)
- Heavy metals: lead, nickel, cadmium, manganese
- Pesticides, herbicides, and insecticides (particularly those containing Carbaryl)
- Fumes from paints, thinners, solvents, wood preservatives, varnishes, glues, spray adhesives, benzene, dry-cleaning fluids, certain plastics, vinyl chloride, rubber tuolene
- Lithium, arsenic
- Contact with cat feces
- PCBs (polychlorinated biphenyl)

And beware of the risks of:

- Incompatible Rh factors (possibly mitigated by one gram vitamin C with bioflavonoids taken daily during the last thirty weeks of pregnancy)
- Amniocentesis
- Electronic Fetal Monitoring, either indirect (ultrasound) or direct (electrode)
- Ultrasound in any form
- Prolonged exposure to extremely high temperatures
- Emmenagogues (see pages 9-10), especially during the first and last trimesters
- Common cooking herbs which may encourage miscarriage: *Basil, Caraway seeds, Celery seed, Ginger, fresh Horseradish, Savory, Marjoram, Nutmeg, Rosemary, Saffron, Sage, Parsley, Tarragon, Thyme, Watercress* (avoid during the first trimester; use sparingly thereafter)
- *Golden Seal root* (stresses liver and kidneys, raises white blood cell count, and can cause uterine contractions)

References and Resources

- *Healing Yourself*
  Joy Gardener; 1982, Box 752, Vashon, WA 98070

- *Lunaception*
  Louise Lacey; 1975, Coward, McCann, and Geoghegan, Inc.
  PO Box 489, Berkeley, CA 94701

- *Hygieia*
  Jeannine Parvati; 1977, Freestone

- *The Use of Herbal Birth Control among Indian Women of North America*
  Barbara Kean; 1977, unpublished paper

- *A Cooperative Method of Natural Birth Control*
  Margaret Nofziger; 1976, Book Publishing Company

- *Mental Birth Control*
  Mildred Jackson & Terri Teague; 1973
  POB 656, Oakland, CA 94604

- *The Natural Birth Control Book;* Art Rosenblum
  Aquarian Research Foundation
  5260 Morton St.
  Philadelphia, PA 19144

- *Conscious Conception*
  Jeannine Parvati Baker, Frederick Hamilton Baker, and Tamara Slayton; 1985, Freestone & Wingbow, co-publishers

- *When Birth Control Fails*
  Suzanne Gage; Speculum Press

- *Using Plants to Induce Miscarriage*
  AlexSandra Lett; 1977
  POB 430, Yellow Springs, OH 45387

- "How Chemicals are Harming Our Genes"
  (includes coffee & tobacco)
  CoEvolution Quarterly, Spring 1979 ($3)
  POB 428, Sausalito, CA 94966

- "Terata: A Mother's Prenatal Health Advisory"
  Mother Jones, January 1985 (reprint $1.55)
  1663 Mission St., San Francisco, CA 94103

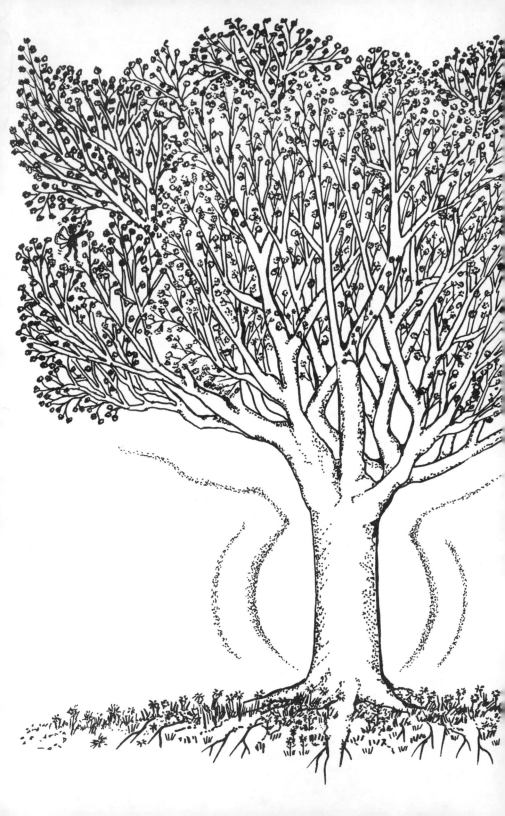

During Pregnancy

Wise Woman healing teaches the importance of excellent nutrition during pregnancy, understanding that you form your child and yourself from the nourishment you receive in the forty weeks of pregnancy. Excellent nutrition includes pure water, controlled breath, abundant light, loving and respectful relationships, beauty and harmony in daily life, positive, joyous thoughts, and vital foodstuffs.

Wise Women see that most of the problems of pregnancy can be prevented by attention to nutrition. Morning sickness and mood swings are connected to low blood sugar; backaches, hypertension, and severe labor pains often result from insufficient calcium; varicose veins, hemorrhoids, constipation, skin discoloration, and anemias are evidence of lack of specific nutrients; pre-eclampsia, the most severe problem of pregnancy, is a form of acute malnutrition.

Be aware that during pregnancy you create the cells needed to form two extra pounds of uterine muscle, the nerves, bones, organs, muscles, glands, and skin of your fetus, several pounds of amniotic fluid, a placenta, and a fifty percent increase in your blood volume. In addition, you'll replace many extra kidney and liver cells used to process the waste of two beings instead of one.

Wild foods and organically grown produce, grains, and herbs are the best sources of vitamins, minerals, and other nutrients needed during pregnancy. Get out to gather and grow your own if you can: stretch, bend, breathe, move, touch the earth, take time to talk with the plants and yourself, and open to the delightful play of the fairies.

Tonics During Pregnancy

Tonic herbs improve your general health by balancing and sustaining energy flow and focus in the body. Tonics allay annoyances and prevent major problems. During pregnancy, use wild foods and nourishing tonics to boost your supply of vital minerals and vitamins, increase energy, and improve uterine tone. Some uterine tonics are contraindicated during pregnancy or are restricted to the last few weeks of the pregnancy. But most tonics need to be used regularly, for a tonic is to the cells much like exercise is to the muscles: not much use when done erratically. Of course you will benefit even from occasional use of tonics during pregnancy, since they do contain nourishing factors, but consider that regular use can mean five times a week or every other day or whatever suits your patterns and needs. So why not replace your morning cup of coffee with a rich Nettle infusion? Brew up some Raspberry leaf tea; put it in the refrigerator and drink it instead of soda, wine, or beer. Add wild greens to your diet weekly; make it a special occasion. Wise Women have recommended herbal tonics for childbearing for thousands of years. These herbs are empirically safe and notably effective.

Red Raspberry Leaves

German:
HIMBEERE

French:
FRAMBOISIER

Chinese:
FU·P'EN·TZU

Russian:
MALINA

Also:
BRAMBLE

Brewed as a tea or as an infusion, *Rubus* is the best known, most widely used, and safest of all uterine/pregnancy tonic herbs. It contains fragrine, an *alkaloid* which gives tone to the muscles of the pelvic region, including the uterus itself. Most of the benefits ascribed to regular use of Raspberry leaf tea throughout pregnancy can be traced to the strengthening power of fragrine or to the nourishing power of the vitamins and minerals found in this plant. Of special note are the rich concentration of vitamin C, the presence of vitamin E, and the easily assimilated calcium and iron. Raspberry leaves also contain vitamins A and B complex and many minerals, including phosphorus and potassium.

Benefits of drinking a Raspberry leaf brew before and throughout pregnancy include:

• *Increasing fertility in both men and women*
Raspberry leaf is an excellent fertility herb when combined with Red Clover.

• *Preventing miscarriage and hemorrhage*
Raspberry leaf tones the uterus and helps prevent miscarriage and postpartum hemorrhage from a relaxed or atonic uterus.

• *Easing of morning sickness*
Many woman attest to Raspberry leaves' gentle relief of nausea and stomach distress throughout pregnancy.

• *Reducing pain during labor and after birth*
By toning the muscles used during labor and delivery, Raspberry leaf eliminates many of the reasons for a painful delivery and prolonged recovery. It does not, however, counter the pain of cervical dilation.

• *Providing a safe and speedy parturition*
Raspberry leaf works to encourage the uterus to let go and function without tension. It **does not strengthen contractions** but does allow the contracting uterus to work more effectively and so may make the birth easier and faster.

• *Helping to bring down an undelivered placenta*
Raspberry leaf by itself is not effective for this problem. Combined with Ground Ivy or Angelica it does facilitate the birth of the placenta, but either of those herbs alone would do.

• *Assisting in production of plentiful breast milk*
The high mineral content of Raspberry leaf assists in milk production, but its astringency may counter that for some women.

Nettle Leaves

Less well known as a pregnancy tonic but deserving a wider reputation and use, *Urtica dioica* is one of the finest nourishing tonics known. It is reputed to have more chlorophyll than any other herb. The list of vitamins and minerals in this herb includes nearly every one known to be necessary for human health and growth. Vitamins A, C, D, and K, calcium, potassium, phosphorus, iron, and sulphur are particularly abundant in Nettles. The infusion is a dark green color approaching black. The taste is deep and rich. If you are blessed with a Nettle patch near you, use the fresh plant as a pot herb in the spring. Some pregnant women alternate weeks of Nettle and Raspberry brews; others drink Raspberry until the last month and then switch to Nettles to insure large amounts of vitamin K in the blood for the birth.

Pot herbs are wild or cultivated greens best eaten cooked.

Benefits of drinking Nettle infusion before and throughout pregnancy include:

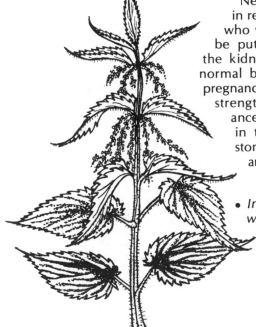

- *Aiding the kidneys*
  Nettle infusions were instrumental in rebuilding the kidneys of a woman who was told that she would have to be put on a dialysis machine. Since the kidneys must cleanse 150% of the normal blood volume for most of the pregnancy, Nettle's ability to nourish and strengthen them is of major importance. Any accumulation of minerals in the kidneys, such as gravel or stones, is gently loosened, dissolved and eliminated by the consistent use of Nettle infusions.

- *Increasing fertility in men and women*

- *Nourishing mother and fetus*

- *Easing leg cramps and other muscle spasms*
- *Diminishing pain during and after birth*

The high calcium content, which is readily assimilated, helps diminish muscle pains in the uterus, in the legs, and elsewhere.

German:
GROSSE BRENESSEL

- *Preventing hemorrhage after birth*

Nettle is a superb source of vitamin K, and increases available hemoglobin, both of which decrease the likelihood of postpartum hemorrhage. But the effectiveness is hard to prove—if it works, nothing happens! Fresh Nettle juice, in teaspoon doses, slows profuse postpartum bleeding.

French:
GRANDE ORTIE,
ORTIE DIOIQUE

Chinese:
HSIEH·TZU·TS'AO

Russian:
KRAPIVA

Also:
STINGING NETTLE

- *Reducing hemorrhoids*

Nettle's mild astringency and general nourishing action tightens and strengthens blood vessels, helps maintain arterial elasticity, and improves venous resiliency.

- *Increasing the richness and amount of breast milk.*

Calcium

Of course calcium is a mineral, not an herbal tonic, but it is so important during pregnancy and throughout our woman lives that I consider it a tonic. Lack of adequate calcium during pregnancy is associated with muscle cramps, backache, high blood pressure, intense labor and afterbirth pains, osteoporosis, tooth problems, and pre-eclampsia.

Calcium assimilation is governed by exercise, stress, acidity during digestion, availability of vitamins C, A, and especially D, and availability of magnesium and phosphorus in the body and diet. Getting the 1000-2000 mg of calcium you need every day of your pregnancy (and life) is not hard with the help of Wise Woman herbs.

- Best food sources of calcium are fish and dairy products, but there is controversy about the assimilation of calcium from pasteurized, homogenized milk. My preferred food sources include **goat milk** and goat milk cheese, salmon, **sardines,** mackerel, **seaweed** (especially kelp), sesame salt (gomasio), tahini, and dark leafy greens such as turnip tops, beet greens, and kale.

● There are roughly 200 grams of calcium in two ounces of nuts (excluding peanuts), one ounce of dried seaweed, two ounces of carob powder, one ounce of cheese, half a cup of cooked greens (kale, collards, Dandelion especially), half a cup of milk, three eggs, four ounces of fish, or one tablespoon of molasses.

● Most **wild greens** are exceptionally rich in calcium and the factors needed for calcium's absorption and use. Lamb's Quarters, Mallow, Galinsoga, Shepherd's Purse, Knotweed, Bidens, Amaranth, and Dandelion leaves all supply more calcium per 100 grams than milk.

● Bones soaked in apple cider vinegar release their calcium into the acidic vinegar. A tablespoonful of this vinegar in a glass of warm water supplies needed calcium and is good for morning sickness too!

● Many fruits are rich in calcium (though not as rich as the above foods). Dried dates, figs, raisins, prunes, papaya and elderberries are the best sources.

● **Raspberry leaf infusion** contains calcium in its most absorbable form. Assimilation is further enhanced by the presence of phosphorus and vitamins A and C in the Raspberry leaves.

● **Fresh Parsley** and **Watercress** are available in most grocery stores year-round. They are both good sources of many minerals and vitamins, including calcium, phosphorus, vitamin A, and vitamin C.

● **Nettle infusions** supply calcium and phosphorus, vitamin A and the vital vitamin D, in a readily assimilated form.

● Avoid these foods which are thought to interfere with the absorption of calcium: spinach, chocolate, rhubarb, and brewer's yeast.

● Do not use bone meal or oyster shell tablets as sources of supplemental calcium. They have been found to be high in lead, mercury, cadmium, and other toxic metals.

Late Pregnancy Tonics

• **Squaw Vine leaves**   A tea (not infusion) or tincture of *Mitchella repens* is considered safe and helpful during the last 4-6 weeks of pregnancy. The usual dosage is two cups of tea daily, or 20-30 drops of tincture in a cup of Raspberry leaf tea (or water) twice a day. Some midwives use Squaw Vine only when uterine "weakness" is indicated by irregular periods, or bleeding during the first trimester. Healthy, full term, no problem pregnancies are the result.

• **Blue/Black Cohosh roots**   *Caulophyllum thalictroides* and *Cimicifuga racemosa* are safely used as teas or tinctures only during the last 4-6 weeks of pregnancy, not before. The usual dosage is 5-10 drops of each tincture in a cup of water twice daily, or up to two cups of tea a day. The Cohoshes work "synergistically, not interchangeably," according to one midwife, who stresses the importance of combination use. Another midwife reports precipitous labor when Blue Cohosh is taken alone or with Pennyroyal during the last six weeks of pregnancy. See page 65 for more information on the Cohoshes.

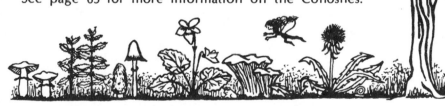

Tonics to Avoid

• **PN6 Capsules**   Several women and midwives report that the use of PN6, even as a tea, causes problems such as early contractions when taken 4-6 weeks before the due date.

• **False Unicorn and Dong Quai**   These tonic roots are considered too powerful in their effect on the uterus to be used during pregnancy without professional advice.

Problems During Pregnancy

Morning Sickness

Nausea and mild vomiting in the morning during the first trimester of pregnancy is a common problem, for which there are many remedies. Most *allopathic* anti-nausea medicines contain antihistamines, which have been shown to cause birth defects in animals. The following herbal and "old wives'" preventions and remedies have no known harmful side effects. If the morning sickness persists beyond the third month of the pregnancy, seek the assistance of a Wise Woman.

Preventing Morning Sickness

• There is a strong connection between nausea in early pregnancy and low **blood sugar.** Maintain your blood sugar level by eating small meals frequently (even every few hours) and by eating a protein-rich snack, such as popcorn with nutritional yeast, or brown rice with miso, or bread and tahini, before going to sleep.

• Chemical by-products of the increased hormonal activity of pregnancy, if allowed to build up in the body, can cause morning sickness. **Walk** a mile a day to prevent this.

• Increase available **iron** and the **vitamin B complex** (especially B_1 and B_6) through diet or supplements. A vitamin B_6 deficiency may cause morning sickness; supplements of 10-20 mg daily will completely relieve this nausea. See Appendix I for herbal sources of iron and B complex.

• Eat unsalted crackers or matzo before getting out of bed.

• Avoid spicy and greasy foods; even cooking greasy foods for someone else may nauseate you.

• Get out of bed slowly in the morning avoiding any sudden movements.

• Drink a cup of **Anise** or **Fennel** seed tea when you wake up.

• Drink one teaspoon of apple cider vinegar in 8 ounces of warm water first thing in the morning.

Remedies for Morning Sickness

The following remedies are listed in order of increasing strength. The mildest remedies are often sufficient, so try those first.

• Open the window or go outside to get some **fresh air.**

• Drink a cup or two of **Raspberry leaf** tea or infusion each day. Sipping the infusion before getting up or sucking on ice cubes made from the infusion increases the strength of this remedy.

• Try any one of these *homeopathic* remedies: Ipecac 30x, Nux vomica 6x, Cannabis 30x.

• Drink a tea made from dried Peach tree leaves to help control morning sickness distress.

• Sip **Peppermint** or **Spearmint** infusion first thing in the morning. This is a stimulating eye-opener and effective anti-nauseant.

• Take tablespoonful doses of **Ginger** root tea anytime nausea occurs. It is especially effective for motion sickness and early morning queasiness.

★ Wild Yam root   *Dioscorea villosa* is specific and powerful for nausea of pregnancy. It is slower to work, but more effective and far safer than Bendectin, the allopathic medicine. Take sips of the infusion throughout the day. Or take teaspoonfuls of the decoction several

Aztec:
CHIPAHUACXIHUITL
"graceful plant"

times daily. Or use a dropperful of the tincture in a glass of water or Mint tea once or twice a day.

● Ginger root   Powdered and encapsulated, *Zingiber officinale* is taken in doses of up to 25 capsules per day for complete control of severe nausea and vomiting throughout pregnancy.

Visualization for Morning Sickness

When morning sickness is severe or chronic, visualization can be used to give access to emotional aspects of the problem. Sit quietly and allow your mind to bring up images connected with the vomiting/nausea. What can't you stomach? What do you want to clear out? What don't you accept? Examine and acknowledge each image as it arises, then let it float away or dissolve. We are complex beings, capable of desiring and despising simultaneously; allow yourself to see what it is about the pregnancy that makes you want to throw up. Repeat the visualization once or twice a day for at least a week for best results.

Miscarriage

Twenty percent of all pregnant women miscarry, usually during the first trimester. The most common causes of miscarriage are 1) herbicides, pesticides, radiation, etc. in your water, air, and food, 2) loose or "incompetent" os, and 3) hormonal imbalances. Herbal remedies cannot correct the first two causes. They may be helpful, however, in preventing miscarriages due to hormonal imbalances. Herbal remedies may also be used to complete a miscarriage and control bleeding. The general experience is that miscarriage is not preventable once bright red blood shows. (CAUTION: If bleeding occurs as a continuous flow anytime in the last three months, a life-threatening emergency may exist.) "Old wives' tales" have it that these herbal remedies will not stop the miscarriage if it is occurring due to fetal abnormality or severe misplacement of the placenta. The listings are in order of increasing strength.

Preventing Chronic Miscarriage

• Attention to correct nutrition and lifestyle habits (no coffee, tobacco, or alcohol) is especially important for women who have a history of miscarriage.

• The inverted yoga postures—headstand and shoulder stand—are recommended for women carrying twins who are threatening to make an early appearance.

• **Black Haw root bark**   *Viburnum prunifolium* is regarded as an especially effective miscarriage preventative. Begin drinking one or two cups of tea or a half cup of the infusion daily as soon as you are pregnant. Black Haw may be used throughout the entire pregnancy if desired.

• **False Unicorn root**   *Chamaelirium luteum* is strongly recommended for women who have experienced repeated miscarriages. It may be of help even when the cervix is too loose to hold the pregnancy, as it is a powerful tonic. Use 3 drops of the tincture four to five times daily, beginning a month before conception and continuing for the entire first trimester.

Preventing Threatened Miscarriage

• Bed rest, relaxation, and vitamin E (up to 2000 IU a day during the crisis period) are strongly recommended when miscarriage threatens.

• Alcohol (for example, whiskey) relaxes the smooth muscles and can be used to slow or stop uterine contractions if sipped when cramping is felt. Intravenous alcohol is still used in hospitals to help forestall threatened miscarriages.

• **Wild Yam root**   The source material for hormonal birth control pills, *Dioscorea villosa* contains glycosides from which the body can manufacture the hormones progesterone and cortisone, which are needed to maintain a pregnancy. The infusion is the strongest

Also:
COLIC ROOT, CHINA
ROOT, RHEUMATISM
ROOT

preparation; take 2-4 ounces every half hour for threatened miscarriage. Results should be evident by the second dose. The tincture is less effective and may cause nausea or vomiting; use 10 drops every half hour as needed.

Also:
ASTHMA WEED,
GAGROOT, PUKE WEED,
WILD TOBACCO,
EMETIC WEED

● **Lobelia herb**   Indian Tobacco is another name for *Lobelia inflata*, which is said to aid the miscarriage if the fetus is weak or malformed, but prevent it if the fetus is strong and healthy. Take the leaf and seed tea in sips every few minutes throughout a full hour; after an hour's rest, repeat. Lobelia tea causes nausea or vomiting in some women. The tincture is usually less nauseating. Take no more than 15 drops in a small glass of water, as often as every fifteen minutes, for several days if needed.

● For bleeding near term (possible abruption of the placenta) take:
   1,500 IU vitamin E (3 doses of 500 IU)
   50,000 IU vitamin A (2 doses of 25,000 IU)
   6,000 mg vitamin C (6 doses of 1,000 mg)
   50 mg zinc (with food)
daily for up to two weeks, or until the pregnancy is stabilized. Midwives claim that the vitamin E glues the placenta back on and holds it until the pregnancy achieves full term. CAUTION: Large doses of vitamin E taken within one week of term may cause abnormal adhesion of the placenta after the birth.

● Threatened Miscarriage Brew - See Appendix II

Completing a Miscarriage

BLACK COHOSH
Also:
BLACK SNAKEROOT,
COHOSH BUGBANE,
BATTLEWEED,
RATTLETOP,
RICHWEED

Russian:
KLOPOGON DAURSKY

● To complete a miscarriage, 1) have an experienced and skilled assistant with you, 2) have herbs which control bleeding on hand, and 3) use 20 drops each of Blue and Black Cohosh tinctures every hour to empty the uterus. Do not exceed five doses.

● To control bleeding, use 10-20 drops of Shepherd's Purse tincture or Witch Hazel tincture (not drugstore variety) under the tongue as often as needed. (See pages 71-73.)

Varicose Veins/Hemorrhoids

A tendency to varicosities (weak or broken spots in the veins) in the rectum (hemorrhoids) and in the legs, groin and vulva (varicose veins) is often inherited. Ask your grandmothers, mother, and sisters if they were bothered during or after their pregnancies and if they were, be especially careful not to stress your body by long periods of standing or constipation. Even if they weren't, take care of your circulatory and eliminatory systems as preventative maintenance. The increased blood volume during pregnancy stresses the veins, and the heightened levels of progesterone (normal during pregnancy) relax the smooth muscles and impair venous return of the blood; both things make varicosities more likely. Sometimes varicosities don't appear until after the delivery; it is not unusual to suddenly have huge hemorrhoids two or three days after giving birth. Commercial preparations such as Preparation H, Americaine, and Anusol should not be used for hemorrhoids during pregnancy because they contain local anesthetics and mercury which are absorbed through the skin and can be harmful to the fetus. These herbal remedies, including exercise and diet, prevent and deal safely with varicosities, whether you experience them before, during, or after your pregnancy.

Exercise for Varicosities

★ **Leg inversions** help prevent varicose veins, backaches and muscle cramps. Lie on your back on the floor, propping your lower legs up on a couch, chair, or bed, and bending the knees. Relax for 10-15 minutes, then stand and gently slap up and down your legs with open palms.

• Inverted yoga postures—headstand, plow, shoulder stand—relieve the pressure on the lower veins. They are best done with expert guidance, especially during the last months.

• **Swimming** and brisk **walking** are excellent exercises for the circulatory system; both aid digestion and help keep the bowels working regularly.

Also for Varicosities

• **Support stockings,** while not a replacement for exercise, are useful if your life requires a lot of standing and you have a tendency toward varicose veins. Raise your legs up high for a while before putting the stockings on.

• A five minute leg **massage** daily feels great and does wonders. Work up, with the flow of the veins, and work hard and deep.

• **Avoid:** tight clothing, knee-high stockings, crossing your legs, sitting in one position for a long time (like in the car), high heeled shoes, and straining at the toilet.

Diet for Varicosities

• **Raw garlic, onions** and **lecithin** (especially the liquid form) help veins maintain or regain elasticity. Eat them daily.

• Okra, buckwheat, oats, wheat germ, and **green leafy vegetables** nourish and strengthen the entire circulatory system.

• Foods rich in vitamins A, C, E, and B complex (B_6 for hemorrhoids) are recommended for all circulatory problems.

• **Rutin,** found naturally in association with vitamin C, is specific for repairing broken capillaries. Buckwheat, Rue, and Elder leaves are notable sources of rutin. CAUTION: Do not take rutin tablets during the first trimester.

• **Beets,** grated and steamed, cleanse the liver and promote easy elimination, thus relieving stress on hemorrhoids.

• Vitamin E supplements are helpful in preventing and reducing varicosities; up to 600 IU daily is considered safe during pregnancy.

• **Avoid** all spices, especially Cayenne and Black Pepper and hot sauces and curries. These increase congestion in the offending veins, often causing bleeding from the hemorrhoids.

Herbs for Varicosities

• **Oatstraw** tea or infusion is useful to strengthen the capillaries. Drink one or two cups daily; there is no known overdose.

• **Nettle** leaf infusion improves the elasticity of the veins. Use at least one cup per day throughout pregnancy and lactation.

• **Parsley** raw or as a tea is beneficial to the veins. Use it abundantly in salads or drink up to a half cup of tea daily.

• **Avoid** internal use of Aloe vera products, and tea of Yellow or White Sweet Clover, as these herbs draw blood to the lower half of the body and can increase the problem. (Red Clover tea doesn't.)

First Aid for Varicose Veins

• Apply **Witch Hazel** (from the drugstore) with a plant mister or a saturated cloth. The astringency is pain relieving and helps tighten the tissues and reduce the swelling.

• Prepare an infusion or fresh poultice of **Comfrey, Yarrow,** or **Mullein** leaves and apply as a compress to ease achiness and tighten veins.

• Wash varicosities with **Oak bark** infusion or apple cider vinegar to soothe pain.

First Aid for Hemorrhoids

• Apply **baking soda**, wet or dry, to take away the itch. (This may feel hot or burning for a short while.)

- Try homeopathic **Hamamelis 30x.**

- Apply lemon juice or **drugstore Witch Hazel** to reduce swelling and curb bleeding. (This will sting.)

- Apply grated raw potato to ease swelling and pain.

- Apply **Comfrey** or **Yellow Dock root ointment** to reduce swelling, stop bleeding, and ease pain.

- Insert a peeled clove of Garlic (which may be wrapped in one layer of gauze and oiled) into the rectum overnight to minimize swelling.

- Use a **Plantain and Yarrow ointment** to relieve pain immediately and to shrink hemorrhoids within a few days. This combination salve has restored normalcy to some women who have been incapacitated for years.

- Eliminate even severely swollen, protruding and bleeding hemorrhoids with **herbal sitz baths.** Witch Hazel is indisputably the best herb for this, but Plantain leaves, Comfrey root, White Oak bark, Sea Grape leaves/bark or other strong *astringents* may be substituted. Prepare an infusion of the herb, making 8 cups (4 oz. of dried herb in a half gallon of boiling water, steeped for 8 hours). Separate the liquid from the herbs and pour it into a shallow basin or pan. Sit in this for 15 minutes at least twice a day. Don't worry about getting every hemorrhoid wet; the herbs are absorbed through the skin and work their magic without direct contact. Most people experience pain relief with the first sitz bath, and the hemorrhoids often shrink and disappear within a few days. This may be repeated as often as you desire, using the same liquid over and over.

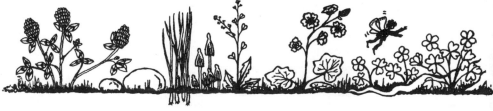

Constipation

One of the changes of pregnancy is a slowing of the action of the intestinal tract which makes constipation (hard and infrequent stools) more likely. Stresses such as emotional upheavals or changes in diet and sleep patterns can also lead to constipation. Constipation during pregnancy often comes from taking allopathic iron supplements such as ferrous sulphate. Iron from herbal sources, such as Yellow Dock root, is rarely constipating. Commercial and herbal laxatives should not be used during pregnancy.

Preventing Constipation

• Replace refined white flour products such as bread, noodles, cookies, cakes, bagels, donuts, pizza, pancakes, and pretzels with **whole grain** products such as bran muffins, whole wheat bread, brown rice, tortillas, oatmeal, and popcorn.

• Increase your liquid intake by eating soups, shakes (homemade with honey, fresh fruit, and yogurt), fruit and vegetable juices (fresh if possible), and herbal teas between meals.

• **Eat less red meat,** especially smoked and cured meat like bacon, ham, sausage, and pastrami.

• **Exercise.** Walking, swimming, and yoga are invaluable in preventing any number of discomforts of pregnancy, including constipation.

• My mother's favorite preventative: set aside a regular time every day to have a bowel movement. Rushing to go to work or do errands without taking time for eating and eliminating often result in constipation. Elimination normally follows the morning meal within half an hour. If you are pressed for time, you can prompt your body to have a bowel movement by stimulating your lips and tongue with your teeth or by drinking a cup of hot herbal tea on an empty stomach.

Remedies for Constipation

● Take **bran** with plenty of water. Widely recommended for preventing constipation, bran can actually cause it by absorbing liquid in the intestines and hardening the stool.

● Drink **prune juice** and eat prunes for gentle and safe softening of the feces. Rhubarb, figs, and maple syrup also open the bowels and relieve constipation.

● Most **fresh greens** are laxative and rich in minerals. **Amaranth,** Lamb's Quarter, and Violet leaves are especially recommended. Cook them or dry and make an infusion.

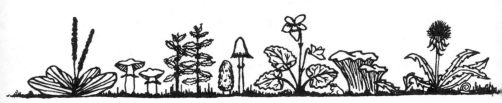

Skin Discoloration

Brownish patches called cloasma, or melasma, or mask of pregnancy, may appear on your face (forehead, upper lip, cheeks) during pregnancy or while taking birth control pills. This discoloration usually disappears after the birth, but may linger for years after discontinuing the Pill. There is a link between cloasma and elevated levels of certain hormones; there is also a connection with deficiencies of folic acid and PABA.

Preventing Skin Discoloration

● Cloasma may appear or worsen considerably after exposure to sunlight. A PABA sunscreen, a big brimmed hat, or frequently coating the face with St. John's/Joan's Wort oil will decrease this possibility. (See St. Joan's Wort Oil—Appendix II.)

● Foods rich in PABA and folic acid include nutritional yeast, molasses, wheat germ, whole grains, liver, mushrooms, fresh fruits, and fresh vegetables.

Folic Acid Anemia

• Folic acid is a component of the vitamin B complex. It works best in combination with vitamins C and B₁₂. Folic acid is rapidly destroyed by heat and light. As it is scarce even in the best sources, try to include one of these herbs or foods at every meal if you are deficient, as indicated by your prenatal blood work.

Folic/Folia
Find Folic acid in all green leaves (folia).

• Best herbal sources of folic acid are Watercress, Parsley, Chicory, Dandelion, Amaranth, and Lamb's Quarter greens.

• Best food sources of folic acid are whole grains, liver, and leafy greens.

• CAUTION: Epileptics should be cautious about pill supplements of folic acid; doses over 1 mg daily may increase seizures.

Iron Deficiency Anemia

Iron is found in every cell of the body, but the amount present is most easily calculated from a blood sample. If the hemoglobin count of the blood sample is 12 or less, then a deficiency of iron is said to exist. It is possible that many diagnoses of iron deficiency anemia during pregnancy are a result of misinterpretation of the body's natural physiological changes while pregnant, and that lower hemoglobin levels, especially during the second trimester when the blood volume increases sharply, are normal. Ferrous sulphate is commonly prescribed to prevent and correct iron deficiency anemia during pregnancy. There are many reasons to avoid it: ferrous sulphate is poorly absorbed (only 10-30%); it stresses the organs of elimination (liver, kidneys, intestines) which must process it out of the body; it is very constipating; it may cause indigestion; miscarriages have been associated with its use; and it may irritate the kidneys and cause them to break down. The following herbs have none of these detrimental side effects and work more effectively than ferrous sulphate to raise the hemoglobin level of the blood.

Spanish:
LENGUA DE VACA,
CANAGRIA

Chinese:
CHIN·CH'IAO MAI

Russian:
KONSKY SHAVEL

Also:
CURLY DOCK,
NARROW DOCK,
PATIENCE DOCK,
SOUR DOCK.

Dock leaves make
a good pot herb.

● **Yellow Dock root**   The yellow roots of many *Rumex* species, prepared as a decoction, syrup, or tincture, provide an excellent, fully absorbable, non-constipating source of iron. To prevent anemia, use 1 tablespoon of decoction or 25-40 drops of the tincture daily. If anemia is present, use the same dosage, but take it three times a day. Yellow Dock root is commonly used by herbalists to replenish hemoglobin after a hemorrhage.

● Other herbal sources of iron include Parsley, Nettles, Amaranth greens, Dandelion root, and Kelp. Also see Appendix I.

● Best food sources of iron are liver, leafy greens, beets, oysters, heart, and tongue.

● Vitamin C aids assimilation of iron.

● Avoid coffee, tea, excess bran, alkalinizers, and phosphates; they inhibit absorption of iron.

● Anemia Prevention Brew - See Appendix II.

Muscle/Leg Cramps

Cramping of the muscles in the sides, legs, and feet is an annoying and common occurrence during the latter part of many pregnancies. Lack of calcium is the major culprit, with lack of salt and poor circulation contributing to the problem. There are no safe commercial medicines to take for muscle cramps during pregnancy. A combination of exercise, herbs, and diet is necessary to keep calcium levels high and prevent cramps. (See pages 21-22.)

Exercise to Prevent Muscle Cramps

● Walk or swim as often as possible.

● Take a yoga class or do yoga or stretching exercises at home, but be careful not to point your toes.

• Treat yourself to a full body massage at least once a month.

• Use leg inversions to prevent cramps. See instructions on page 29.

• Stretch the calf muscles with slow lunges. Done before bed, lunges minimize leg and foot cramps during the night. Placing one foot well in front of the other, gradually bend the forward leg at the knee and lean forward. Keep the back leg straight, with the heel flat on the floor. You may balance by placing your hands against a wall.

First Aid for Muscle Cramps

• Leg cramps: sit on floor, straighten leg with cramp, pull toes toward body.

• Foot cramps: roll foot over a bottle about three inches in diameter. If your feet cramp during the night, keep the bottle under your bed for easy access.

• All muscle cramps respond to warm moist heat.

Backache

The increasing weight of the growing fetus, movements of a body whose center of gravity has shifted, stress on the kidneys, and the difficulty of sitting in and arising from chairs and beds contribute to backaches throughout pregnancy. There are no medications, not even aspirin, which are safe to take during pregnancy to prevent or relieve backaches. Painful backaches can be forestalled and relieved with exercise, intelligent food selection, and wise use of herbs. Strong abdominal muscles, firm beds, and hard chairs will support the growing fetal weight and take the pressure off the back. Good posture and regular exercise will establish the new center of gravity. Herbs can nourish and strengthen the kidneys.

Exercise for Backache

• **Cat/Cow** can be practiced daily or whenever needed. Get on your hands and knees on a firm surface; inhale, let your head hang down and arch your back up like a cat; exhale, lift your head all the way up and let your spine return to parallel with the floor. Continue flexing the spine up and down while breathing rhythmically. This exercise can also be done in a standing position.

• **Knee/Chest Twists** stretch the spine and keep it supple. Once a day, or when needed, lie on your back on a firm surface and pull your knees to your chest. Stretch your arms straight out to the sides. Roll your knees to the left and your head to the right; relax for half a minute, then roll your knees to the right and your head to the left and relax again. Repeat once or twice.

Also for Backache

• Chiropractic adjustments are one of the best preventatives of backache during pregnancy.

• Sleep with pillows supporting your legs, back and belly.

• Be especially careful to lift heavy objects by bending your knees, not your back.

• Wear shoes which have flat heels and offer good support to the feet and legs.

Diet for Backache

• Minerals needed to diminish and prevent backache include calcium and magnesium. Refer to pages 21-22 for best sources of calcium. Magnesium is found in all fresh green vegetables, apples, figs, wheat germ, and all seeds and nuts, especially almonds.

• Lemon juice in water, up to six glasses daily, benefits the kidneys, easing backache.

Herbs for Backache

• **Wheat grass juice** is highly recommended for all ills, including backaches. The bright green juice of the wheat sprouts contains a plentiful supply of the nutrients needed to strengthen muscles, ease the nerves, and keep the spine flexible. To prepare the juice: soak wheat berries overnight, drain off the water, and spread the wheat one berry deep onto an inch thick layer of dirt on a cookie sheet with edges. Water the whole thing several times a day. Harvest the green shoots by cutting them when they are several inches high. Use a special wheat grass juicer to extract the most juice, or blend the shoots with water in your blender, then strain and drink the liquid.

Learn more about wheat grass from Dr. Ann Wigmore at Hippocrates Health Institute in Boston, Mass.

• **Nettle** infusion is unsurpassed for toning and aiding kidneys.

• **Comfrey** infusion provides every vitamin and mineral necessary to prevent backaches. It is also rich in amino acids, the building blocks of protein, needed in plentiful supply for strong abdominal muscles and healthy babies.

• See Appendix I for herbal sources of calcium, magnesium, vitamins C, D, E, and B complex, all needed when backache is a problem.

First Aid for Backache

• Heat—a warm bath, a hot shower, a hydroculator, a hot water bottle, a towel dipped in boiling water—will provide temporary relief for most backaches.

• Tiger Balm, Olbas, Zheng Gu Shui, Wintergreen oil and other homemade or purchased **herbal liniments** and rubs can penetrate into deep muscle tissue to relieve tension and pain. They work best if followed by moist heat.

• St. John's/Joan's Wort   *Hypericum perforatum* is highly effective at relieving backaches. The tincture is a specific for muscle spasms; use 15-25 drops in a glass of water every few hours as needed. For severe pain, add 3-5 drops of Skullcap tincture. The infused oil of St. J's has the

Spanish: TENCHALITA

German: JOHANNISKRAUT

French:
HERBE DE ST. JEAN,
MILLEPERTUIS PERFORE

Russian:
ZVEROBOI

unique ability to enter the nerve endings, relieving pain
and easing any nervous system irritation. It works like a
chiropractic adjustment, but through a different route: the
nerve endings are soothed and the muscle relaxes; once
the muscle is released, the vertabrae slide back into place.
(See Appendix II for instructions on making St.
John's/Joan's Wort tincture and oil.)

Heartburn

This is the common name for the sensation of pain, heat,
and acidic burning in the esophagus experienced after
eating. It may be caused by nervous tension, excess
production of stomach acids, relaxed stomach muscles
which allow foods to back up, or the mechanical
displacement of the stomach by the upward movement of
the enlarging uterus. It is most common during the last
half of the pregnancy. The numerous commercial
remedies for heartburn (such as Alka-Seltzer, Rolaids,
baking soda and other antacids) are contraindicated
during pregnancy. The following remedies are considered
safe and effective for pregnant women.

Preventing Heartburn

• Eat small meals frequently. Take a bag of nuts and dried
fruit with you when you are away from home.

• Chew, chew, chew! And eat slowly.

• Don't drink while eating; do consume plenty of liquids
between meals. If you must drink with meals, try half a
lemon squeezed into a glass of water.

• Notice which foods seem to produce your heartburn
and eliminate them from your diet. Greasy and highly
seasoned foods are a problem for many women.

• Be aware that coffee and cigarettes increase heartburn
by irritating the stomach.

• Avoid lying down after eating.

• Make **Anise** or **Fennel** seed tea your after meals or during meals beverage. These seed teas are tonic to the stomach and gently assist digestion.

• Chew on or eat some organic orange peel a few minutes after your meal to aid digestion.

• Eat a small amount of apple peels, pineapple, or, best of all, **papaya** after meals. All forms—fresh, dried, canned, juice, even tablets—contain digestive enzymes.

Remedies for Heartburn

• Sip **yogurt,** cream, or milk to relieve heartburn due to overproduction of stomach acids.

• **Fly** to help the stomach settle down: sit cross-legged and raise and lower your arms quickly, bringing the backs of your hands together over your head.

• Carry raw **almonds** when you travel; chew them slowly to relieve heartburn.

• Slippery Elm   Severe heartburn can usually be allayed by eating a teaspoon of *Ulmus fulva* powder mixed with some honey. Slippery Elm bark neutralizes stomach acids, soothes the stomach, and helps absorb intestinal gas. Slippery Elm throat lozenges, sold in most health food stores, offer a convenient way to use this remedy away from home.

Fatigue and Mood Changes

Hormonal changes, emotional changes, physical changes, and all the attendant stresses of pregnancy may cause extreme fatigue and emotional swings, especially during the last trimester. One midwife advises: "This is the perfect opportunity to touch your own deep emotional truths ... to acknowledge and resolve your inner disharmonies, and to recreate your life as you create another life. The emotional changes experienced during pregnancy are not to be avoided, but valued; they are cathartic and valid." Use exercise, relaxation, meditation, diet, and herbs to improve your energy and moods, but don't neglect emotional and spiritual work.

Feeling Energetic and Peaceful

• Regular moderate exercise combined with affirmations and creative visualizations tones the body and the mind. Ten minutes of exercise done regularly does more to prevent fatigue and depression than an occasional arduous workout.

• **Deep relaxation** is a powerful tool for easing emotional and physical stress. It can be done as a break in the day's demands, just before sleep, or just after waking. See page 62 for a complete relaxation to read or tape.

• **Meditation** refreshes and centers the mind.

• **Affirmations,** visualizations, and forms of active or guided meditation, are important emotional and psychic tools, and are easy to use. Check the resource listing at the end of this chapter for self-help guides to learning and using these skills.

• Indulgence (of yourself, not your obsessions) helps prevent fatigue and depression. Give yourself time to read and relax and create and be easy. Take a stern stand with your guilt about keeping the house clean, or making breakfast for everyone, or excelling at your work, or whatever you ride yourself about. There will be plenty to do when the baby is born; don't exhaust yourself now.

Diet and Herbs for Even Emotions

• Your body's need for minerals and proteins soars during pregnancy. Lack of either registers as a craving for sweets.

Eating sugar may cause blood sugar swings, fatigue, and depression. Eliminate white sugar, and restrict honey, fructose, maple syrup, etc. Focus on **high protein** snacks, such as nuts, yogurt, popcorn with nutritional yeast, sardines, and cheese.

• **Raspberry leaf infusion** calms; add up to half as much **Peppermint** or **Spearmint** for a lift of spirits and a renewed sense of energy.

• Burdock, Blessed Thistle, and Sarsaparilla are **bitter tonics**. Occasional use helps keep your emotions on an even keel and makes a nice change from your daily Nettle or Raspberry leaf brew.

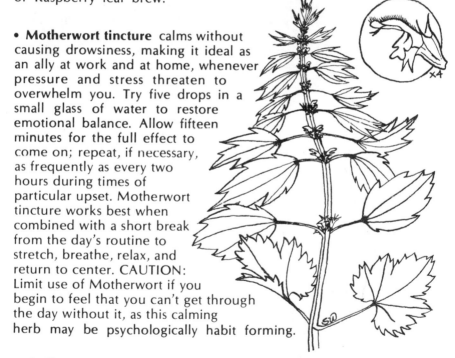

• **Motherwort tincture** calms without causing drowsiness, making it ideal as an ally at work and at home, whenever pressure and stress threaten to overwhelm you. Try five drops in a small glass of water to restore emotional balance. Allow fifteen minutes for the full effect to come on; repeat, if necessary, as frequently as every two hours during times of particular upset. Motherwort tincture works best when combined with a short break from the day's routine to stretch, breathe, relax, and return to center. CAUTION: Limit use of Motherwort if you begin to feel that you can't get through the day without it, as this calming herb may be psychologically habit forming.

• **Skullcap** tincture provides deep, refreshing sleep. Take up to 30 drops of commercial tincture (from dried plants) or 5-15 drops of fresh plant tincture half an hour before you go to bed. An infusion of the dried plant nourishes and strengthens the nerves. Drink two cups daily for several months if your nerves feel frayed and you are easily upset.

Bladder Infections

The blood volume increases 50% during pregnancy. Your kidneys, responsible for cleaning the blood, are called upon to work correspondingly harder, and your entire urinary system becomes more vulnerable to stress and infection. As you enter the last trimester of pregnancy, be alert for warning signs of bladder, or urinary tract, infections: an urgent and frequent impulse to urinate (often with little result), a burning sensation during urination, and a mild aching or cramping in the abdomen. Prompt treatment of early symptoms, and preventative action, are the safest courses for bladder infections during pregnancy, as both herbs and medicines strong enough to cure these infections increase the stress on the kidneys and have other undesirable side effects. Non-symptomatic bladder infections discovered during routine prenatal urine sampling can be successfully treated with the stronger remedies listed last.

Preventing Bladder Infections

• Wear **cotton** underwear or no underwear; avoid tight polyester pants and pantyhose; bacteria thrive in the moist heat trapped by synthetic fibers.

• Drink plenty of **fluids** throughout the day and urinate as soon as you feel the urge; bacteria breed more easily and rapidly in concentrated and held urine.

• Wipe from front to back, and urinate after intercourse; bacteria are easily transferred to the bladder from the rectum and surrounding tissues.

• Avoid bubble bath, bath oil, bath salts; bacterial growth is aided by the resulting change in normal acid/alkaline balance.

• Drink 5-10 cups of **Nettle** tea or infusion every week during the last trimester to strengthen the kidneys.

Remedies for Bladder Infections

• Unsweetened **cranberry juice** can stop a bladder infection that is just developing. The keys to successful use are 1) the juice must not be sweetened at all (no sugar, dextrose, corn syrup, maple syrup, honey, etc.); 2) the juice must be consumed liberally (an 8 ounce glass every hour for ten hours is not excessive); and 3) the juice must be started as soon as the first twinge or suspicion of infection occurs. Buy unsweetened cranberry juice or concentrate in health food stores, or prepare your own "juice" by blending a handful of fresh frozen berries with a cup of water in your blender. Sour!

• **Vitamin C** is helpful in acidifying the urine and "washing" out the bacteria. Doses of up to 500 mg per hour may be used. CAUTION: Large doses of vitamin C may cause loose stools.

★ Uva Ursi   *Arctostaphylos uva-ursi* kills bacteria in the bladder. I have seen it clear up chronic bladder infections resistant to antibiotics and standard allopathic medicines. Because it is a strong diuretic, Uva Ursi requires cautious use during pregnancy. Brew one ounce of Uva Ursi leaves in a quart jar of boiling water for eight hours. Drink one cup of this infusion every twelve hours the first two days, or in severe cases, one cup every four hours. Continue with at least one cup daily for another three days, even if the symptoms disappear sooner. Do not use Uva Ursi for more than ten days.

Spanish:
GAYUBA DE EUROPA,
CORALILLO

German:
BÄRENTRAUBE

French:
RAISIN D'OURS,
BUSSEROLE

Also:
ARBERRY, BEAR-
BERRY, UPLAND
CRANBERRY,
KINNIKINNICK

• Yarrow   The astringency, antibacterial effect, and *diuretic* potency of *Achillea millefolium* is called for if Uva Ursi alone does not clear the bladder infection within five days. Use one half ounce Yarrow flowers and one half ounce Uva Ursi leaves in one quart of boiling water; steep 8 hours. Drink two or three cups daily for no more than five days.

CAUTION: Juniper berries, Horsetail/Shave Grass, and Buchu are contraindicated during pregnancy due to the stress they place on the kidneys.

High Blood Pressure

The two categories of hypertension (high blood pressure) common during pregnancy are chronic hypertension, indicated by consistent blood pressure readings of 130/90 or higher, and gestational hypertension, marked by a steady rise of the blood pressure after the 28th week of gestation. The main danger in both types is to the fetus; blood flow to the placenta is reduced, and necessary oxygen is less available. Gestational hypertension may indicate pre-eclampsia, a severe problem. (See page 49.) The preventative measures listed here can help forestall gestational hypertension and are important aspects of a program of treatment for either type of high blood pressure. The remedies are useful whenever blood pressure is elevated, and are listed in order of increasing strength.

Preventing Hypertension

• **Avoid stimulants** such as spicy or peppery foods, black tea, cola drinks, coffee, nicotine, cocaine, and diet pills.

• Drink **Nettle** or **Raspberry leaf infusions** regularly.

• **Exercise** is one of the best preventatives of high blood pressure. It forces more blood through the veins which then stretch and open up, lowering blood pressure. The most effective exercise works up a sweat and makes the heart pound. Regular exercise done throughout the pregnancy is preferable to a last minute frenzied attempt to lower elevated blood pressure later on.

• Emotional stress can cause temporary or prolonged rises in your blood pressure. It is not so much the emotions which are the stress, but the desire to avoid and deny them which creates conflict with the reality of inner feelings. A safe person or place where you can freely express the confusing, angry, and unhappy aspects of your pregnancy is an important preventative of hypertension.

• Obesity is connected to high blood pressure, but worrying about gaining too much weight may contribute to hypertension as well. A sensible, highly nutritious diet, high in complex carbohydrates and low in processed food, will help prevent excessive gain, worry over weight, and hypertension. Note: Artificially high blood pressure readings can occur if the blood pressure cuff is too small.

Remedies for Hypertension

• Biofeedback, positive affirmations, and visualizations reduce hypertension with utmost safety. Visualize the blood vessels dilating for five minutes several times daily. Affirm: "My blood pressure is now normal." Deep relaxation increases the power of these techniques.

• **Garlic,** Parsley and onions help lower blood pressure. For maximum effect, use large quantities raw. Garlic oil capsules are effective for some women, in doses of 2-10 capsules daily, depending on the severity of the hypertension.

·GARLIC·
Spanish: AJO
French: AIL
Chinese: SUAN
German: KNOBLAUCH
Russian: CHESNOCK

• **Cucumbers** are the food most renowned for reducing high blood pressure. One half cup of cucumber juice or an entire fresh, raw cucumber daily is the suggested amount. Overripe, yellowish ones are the most effective. Cucumbers also relieve constipation and strengthen the kidneys.

• The juice of half a lemon or lime plus two teaspoons of cream of tartar in a half cup water taken once a day for three days safely lowers high blood pressure during pregnancy. If needed, repeat once after a rest of two days.

• Hops   A simple tea of bitter-tasting, sleep-inducing *Humulus lupulus* is strong enough to reduce hypertension and safe enough to take nightly if needed during the last months of pregnancy. CAUTION: Hops is contraindicated for regular use throughout pregnancy, or for use during the first trimester, due to its hormonal precursors.

Spanish: LUPULO
German: HOPFEN
French: HOUBLON GRIMPANT
Chinese: LU·TS'AO
Russian: HMEL
"slightly drunk"

★ **Passionflower**   *Passiflora* species vines are common weeds in the southern areas of North America and well known worldwide as soothers and healers. Midwives report successful control of hypertension using 2-4 capsules of Passionflower daily, or 15 drops of the tincture three times a day. Although blood pressure may return to normal quickly, continue taking Passionflower for several weeks to obtain the most benefit.

★ **Skullcap**   My favorite herb for all problems associated with tension is *Scutellaria lateriflora*. I find the infusion unsurpassed for reducing anxiety and "nerves." Midwives tell me that one or two cups daily reduces high blood pressure during pregnancy. The tincture is not as useful in controlling hypertension.

★ **Hawthorn berries**   A strong and safe *vaso-dilator, Crataegus* species berries work cumulatively and are taken for extended periods for best results. Essential hypertension then, rather than gestational hypertension, is the focus of Hawthorn berry use. The standard preparation is a cold infusion: one ounce of crushed dried berries steeped in two cups of cold water overnight, brought quickly to a boil, strained and taken in sips, one cup per day, every day. The tincture dose is 15 drops, two or three times daily.

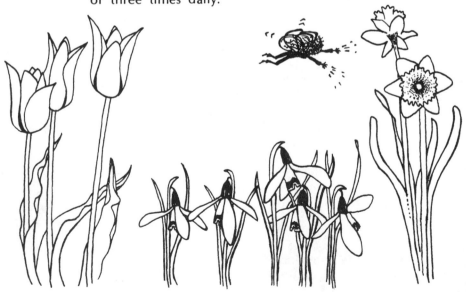

Pre-eclampsia

The most serious and most easily prevented complication of pregnancy is known as metabolic toxemia or pre-eclampsia. The symptoms of pre-eclampsia appear after the 30th week of gestation: *edema*, hypertension, and protein in the urine. Modern medical science does not know the cause of pre-eclampsia. Wise Women see a strong enough connection between deficiencies in the mother's diet and the occurrence of pre-eclampsia to say that pre-eclampsia (and eclampsia, toxemia with maternal convulsions) is the result of malnutrition during pregnancy.

Use the herbal and nutritional information in this section to prevent pre-eclampsia. If you are diagnosed as having pre-eclampsia, use the remedies only in conjunction with the advice of a skilled professional. CAUTION: Poorly managed pre-eclampsia may lead to liver damage or death.

Preventing Pre-eclampsia

• Eat **60-80 grams of protein** daily. Protein is needed to form the growing fetus, uterus, and placenta. There are roughly 25 grams of protein in three cups of milk, or four eggs, or two cups of cooked beans, or two ounces of nuts, or four ounces of fish, meat, or cheese.

• Eat **salt** to taste. Limiting salt during pregnancy does little to prevent swollen ankles and fingers. Lack of adequate salt can cause pre-eclampsia.

• Eat foods high in **calcium.** A study of worldwide eclampsia rates found them to be highest in countries with the lowest calcium intake. **One thousand grams of calcium** daily during pregnancy is a minimum recommendation. (See pages 21-22 for further information on calcium).

• Take in adequate calories. The minimum calorie requirement during pregnancy is **2400 calories a day.**

• Tone and nourish with Raspberry, Nettle, and Dandelion leaves throughout pregnancy. See pages 18-22 and page 51.

Remedies for Pre-eclampsia

• Increase the level of **potassium** in your body. Potassium supplements are a standard part of the allopathic treatment for pre-eclampsia, as they relieve and stabilize some major symptoms of pre-eclampsia: high blood pressure and edema. Potassium is favored by Wise Women because it supports and vitalizes proper functioning of all the organs and systems stressed by pre-eclampsia: liver, kidneys, and nervous system.

Potato peels and bananas are exceptionally rich in potassium; Mint, Chicory, and Dandelion leaves also have extremely high levels of potassium. (Refer to Appendix I for other herbal sources of potassium.)

• Help balance the sodium/potassium ratio of your blood with **raw beet juice,** up to four ounces daily. This is also one of the fastest and most effective ways to increase available calcium in the body. If you don't have access to a vegetable juicer, grate one raw beet and one raw apple together for a satisfying and crunchy snack.

★ Restore the normal balance of sodium and potassium in your body fluids, and promote better functioning of your liver and nervous system by taking 100 mg of vitamin B6 daily in conjunction with a high potency B complex supplement.

★ Augment protein and mineral levels in your body by adding up to three tablespoons of powdered Spirulina or Chorella seaweed to your daily diet.

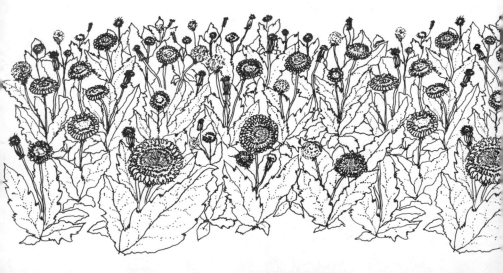

★ *Dandelion leaves*   Easily found in lawns and vacant lots, there are few foods or herbs better for treating pre-eclampsia and strengthening the liver than *Taraxacum*. (Poor functioning of the liver is both symptomatic and causative of pre-eclampsia.)

In addition to vitalizing and healing the liver, Dandelion leaves help the kidneys function better, and are a good source of calcium and potassium. This combination of qualities makes Dandelion leaves a vitally important herb in the prevention and treatment of pre-eclampsia.

Dried Dandelion leaves may be prepared as an infusion, and two or more cups taken daily, but for best results simply eat several ounces of fresh or cooked Dandelion leaves regularly. Three ounces of cooked Dandelion greens contain 12,000 IU vitamin A, 48 mg vitamin C, 140 mg calcium, 230 mg potassium, 1.8 mg iron, choline (essential to the liver), vitamins B$_1$ and B$_2$, and many trace minerals. Have you tried Dandelion greens and found them too bitter for your taste? Do you believe that Dandelion can only be eaten in the spring? Prepared correctly, Dandelion leaves are delicious; they can be picked and eaten year-round. Dandelion Italiano is my favorite recipe. It can be eaten warm or cold, is easily prepared in quantity, and can be stored in the refrigerator for up to two weeks. I have yet to meet a person who dislikes Dandelion leaves prepared this way.

• Dandelion Italiano—See Appendix II.

Spanish:
DIENTE DE LION,
CHICÓRIA

German:
LOWENZAHN,
KUHBLUME

French:
DENT·DE·LION,
PISSENLIT

Russian:
ODUVANCHIK,
PUSHKI

Also:
LION'S TOOTH,
PISS·IN·BED,
WILD ENDIVE,
BLOWBALL,
CONSEUELDA,
FORTUNE TELLER

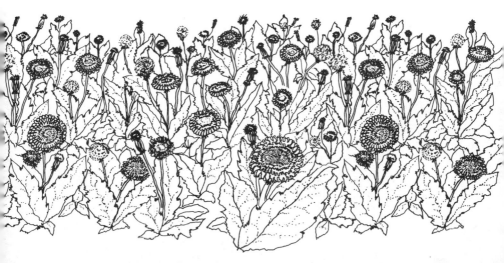

References & Resources

Nutrition:

- *Nutrition Almanac*
  Nutrition Search; 1973, McGraw-Hill

- *Composition of Foods*
  USDA Handbook #8

- *As You Eat So Your Baby Grows*
  Nicki Goldbeck; 1978, Cedar Press

- *How to be a Healthy Mother and Have a Healthy Child*
  Society for the Protection of the Unborn through Nutrition
  SPUN, 17 North Wabash, Suite 603, Chicago, IL 60602

- *The Brewer Medical Diet for Normal and High Risk Pregnancy*
  Gail & Tom Brewer; 1982, Simon and Schuster

Exercises:

- *Essential Exercises for the Childbearing Year*
  Elizabeth Noble; 1976, Houghton Mifflin

- *Prenatal Yoga and Natural Birth*
  Jeanine O'Brien Medvin; 1974, Freestone Pub.

- *Making Love During Pregnancy*
  Libby Coleman; 1977, Bantam Books

Mental and Psychic Skills:

- *Creative Visualization*
  Shakti Gawain; 1978, Whatever Publishing

- *Mother Wit, A Feminist Guide to Psychic Development*
  Diane Meriechild; 1981, The Crossing Press

- *A Gradual Awakening*
  Stephen Levine; 1979, Anchor Books

Remedies:

- *Natural Remedies for Pregnancy Discomforts*
  Free; send stamped, self-addressed, legal size envelope to:
  Department of Consumer Affairs, POB 310, Sacramento, CA 95802

- *The Herb Book*
  John Lust; 1974, Bantam Books

- *The Pregnancy After 30 Workbook*
  Gail Brewer, Ed; 1978, Rodale Press

- *The Handbook of Alternatives to Chemical Medicines*
  Mildred Jackson & Terri Teague; 1975

Also of Interest:

- *Drugs in Pregnancy;* Reba Hill & Leo Stern
- *Environmental Pollution and Pregnancy;* Lawrence Longo, MD
- *Fetal Alcohol Syndrome;* Cheryl Stephens
  Available from March of Dimes Birth Defects Foundation
  1275 Mamaroneck Ave., White Plains, NY 10605

- Coalition for the Medical Rights of Women
  1638 B Haight St., SF, CA 94117

- NAPSAC
  InterNational Association of Parents & Professionals for Safe
  Alternatives in Childbirth; POB 267, Marble Hill, MO 63764

- *Mal(e)Practice*
  Dr. Mendelsohn; 1980, Contemporary Books

- NAG Reports (on pre-eclampsia and nutrition)
  Tom Brewer, MD, #5 Memory Lane, Croton-on-Hudson, NY
  10520

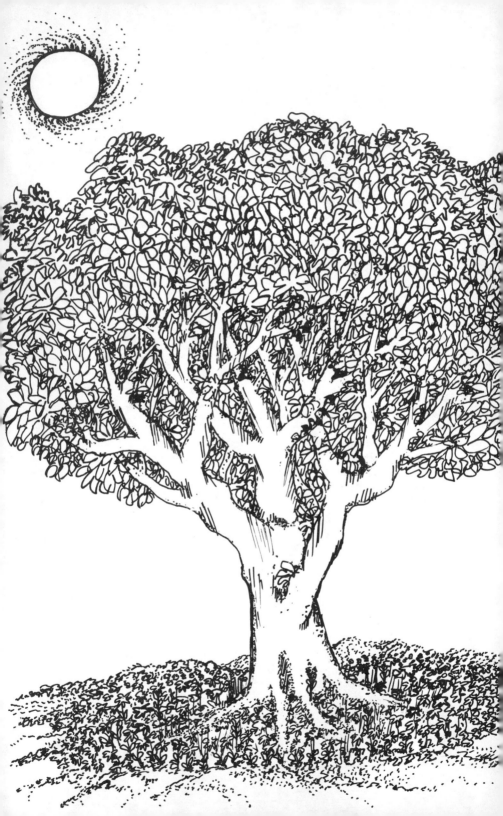

Childbirth

The focal point of the childbearing year, the birth itself, has been in the care of Wise Women in every culture and every time except modern Western civilizations. Our store of wisdom concerning herbs and practices which support and assist all stages of labor has been well preserved and is extensive. What I have compiled here is directed toward your midwife or birth attendant as well as you. Share it with. her/him if you want to avoid drugs during your birth.

Because midwifery is illegal in most states, and use of drugs by unlicensed persons punished severely, many practicing midwives stock their birth bags with herbal allies. I want to thank again these hidden midwives who have contributed their experiences and observations to this Wise Woman Herbal. They remind me to tell you that they find herbs preferable to drugs (though many of them were skeptical at first). They have found that herbs cause fewer side effects in mother and newborn, that the energies of herbs harmonize exceptionally well with the energies of childbirth, and that the incidence of jaundice is much lower in herbal-aided births.

Midwives who rely strictly on drugs for assistance tell me that they "don't want to fool around" with "something that may not work." Understanding their desire to meet emergencies with tried and trusted medicines, I suggest that they experiment with herbs in unstressful circumstances, accumulating understanding of and confidence in herbal remedies before using them at births.

Problems Before Labor

Breech Presentation

Between 20 and 34 weeks, the fetus's position can be ascertained by a skilled midwife or other professional. If the presentation is not head down, these remedies could turn the fetus. It is easier to turn a smaller fetus, so try these remedies early, but remember that before 28-30 weeks the fetus moves around a lot and may undo your effort.

Remedies for Unstable Presentations

★ The most successful do-it-yourself technique for turning a breech fetus is a **headstand** done while totally immersed **in water!** The earlier and more often this is done, the more likely it is to succeed.

• **Postural inversion** is done by lying down with your hips twelve to eighteen inches higher than your shoulders for no more than 20 minutes, two or three times a day. Start at 28 weeks and continue only until the fetus turns and stays head down.

• **Visualization** is an excellent tool for correcting a breech presentation. It need not be time consuming; five minutes of quiet twice a day, during which you envision the fetus lying in your uterus head down, is enough. Remember, in visualizing you try to envision the desired result as already existing, not as becoming or changing. Visualization

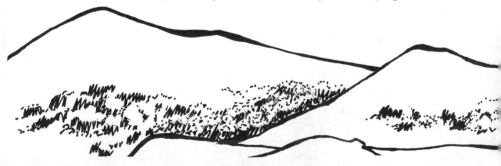

enhances the effect of all other remedies for unstable presentations.

• The homeopathic remedy for unstable presentations is **Pulsatilla 30x.**

• **Swimming** frequently can cause your fetus to turn.

★ Indirect **moxa** (burning Mugwort) on **Bladder 67** (an acupuncture point) can turn a breech presentation. Bladder 67 is on the outside of the little toe on both feet, right next to the nail. Finger pressure may work if moxa is not available. It is best to enlist the aid of someone trained in this technique: acupuncturist, shiatsu therapist, etc.

Pick Mugwort during June's full moon; dry and store it for two years. Then shred fine and form into moxa sticks or cones.

• Before 36 weeks, the fetus may be turned by manipulation from the outside. Properly done, **external version** does not involve pain or force. Seek experienced aid if you wish to use this remedy; heart-tones should be monitored throughout the turning.

False Labor

There is no such thing as "false labor." Early contractions, which may begin up to a week before the birth, are considered helpful by Wise Women who understand the cyclical patterns of birth and who remind us that early labor tunes up the system and tones up the uterus. It is important to eat and sleep regularly if you have early labor. Use the following remedies to ease discomfort when necessary.

• Try a **hot bath and a shot of whiskey** or other spirits just before bedtime if early labor pains keep you awake.

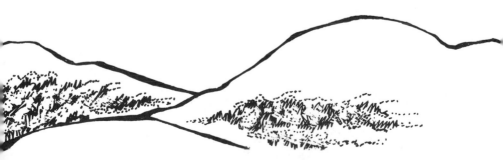

• Ease early labor discomfort with Lobelia tincture. Use a dose large enough to produce relaxation; Lobelia is a stimulant in small doses. Thirty to sixty drops, taken in water once or twice, fifteen minutes apart, is usually effective, and may be repeated as needed.

• Use 5 drops of Motherwort tincture or 25-30 drops of St. Joan's Wort tincture at half-hour intervals to ease the pain of early labor.

• Refer also to Preventing Threatened Miscarriage, pages 27-28.

★ CAUTION: Seek immediate assistance and guidance for premature labor before 37 weeks.

Premature Rupture of Membranes

The breaking of the waters, or membranes, usually occurs after labor is in progress. When it happens before labor has commenced, the risk of infection in the mother and fetus increases greatly. It is assumed that infection becomes more likely as time passes, so allopathic obstetricians in the United States initiate labor after 12-24 hours. But the infection rate in premature babies is also very high, so Wise Woman midwives wait up to two weeks for normal labor to begin. A study by Lewis Mehl showed that premature rupture of membranes (PROM) does increase the risk of infection, but only after four days without labor. If you decide to wait it out, be particularly fastidious about hygiene. Put nothing in your vagina if the membranes are ruptured.

• Try to **outwit all bacteria** looking for warm, dark, moist homes. After toilet use, wipe with "sterilized" toilet paper (bake a roll in a 200° oven for one hour), or rinse off with squirts of water, then pat dry. No baths, no intercourse, no vaginal exams, no free rides for bacteria.

• Supplemental doses of **vitamins C and E** help prevent infection and bleeding.

• Take 5-10 drops of **Echinacea** tincture, two or three times daily as a prophylactic against infection.

• The membranes may reseal spontaneously or with assistance. To encourage resealing lie down immediately. Move as little as possible for 48 hours. Observe and use the power of your thoughts and imagination. Focus on the sensation of the membranes. Visualize the torn edges merged, your amniotic fluid and fetus safely contained within the now whole caul. Drink Nettle, Comfrey, or Violet leaf infusions to encourage the healing. Don't look to see what's happening; be hysterically hygienic.

Unripe Cervix

Before natural labor will begin, your cervix must ripen. Your fingers can tell if your cervix is ripe. An unripe cervix feels like the tip of your nose; as it ripens, it gets softer, more tongue-like. If it is necessary to initiate labor and the cervix is not ripe, these two herbs, together or as simples, will usually hasten the ripening. CAUTION: Do not put your fingers or anything else in the vagina if the membranes are not intact.

French for MIDWIFE sage femme

• Taking **Evening Primrose oil,** three capsules daily for up to a week, may ripen the cervix.

• **Black Cohosh tincture,** 10 drops under the tongue hourly, will have a noticeable effect on the cervix in three or four hours. Continue until the cervix is fully soft and ripe.

★ **Nipple stimulation** is very effective for ripening the cervix and initiating labor. Have someone else suck continually on your nipple, or roll the nipple between your thumb and finger. You may need to continue for many hours to establish regular labor. It's fine to rest during a contraction and resume stimulation as it fades.

Initiating Labor

The herbs used to initiate labor are listed here in order of increasing strength. With the exception of Castor oil (and there is some disagreement on that), these herbs will not be effective unless the cervix is ripe. CAUTION: Do not try to initiate labor unless the fetus is at least 37 weeks gestational age.

• Get the uterus to begin contracting by "imagining" that it is. Don't try to force or push the feeling, just let it arise by itself. If your mind worries or focuses on the problem, gently return yourself to the solution by affirming that labor has begun and that you will feel it very soon. As with all **visualizations,** this one works well with any of the other remedies.

• Homeopathic **Caulophyllum 200x,** is reported as a good labor initiator. The dose can be repeated every half-hour for two hours.

• Labor can be initiated by stimulating the uterus. Rub the belly softly and persistently, with or without oil. Make an infusion of Blue Cohosh and use it as an enema. Have an orgasm. Rub and gently pinch the nipples. All are safe and effective ways to encourage uterine contractions.

★ **Castor oil,** a favorite herbal remedy of Edgar Cayce, is used internally and externally to stimulate the uterus, soften the cervix, and help initiate labor.

Rub Castor oil on the belly and cover with a warm towel if the cervix is ripe and labor seems near.

Or use Castor oil as a stimulating *purgative.* The dosage and procedure for starting labor with Castor oil varies considerably from midwife to midwife, but everyone uses some form of this treatment. Two ounces of Castor oil, two ounces of vodka, and two or more ounces of orange juice is the usual dose. This is often followed with a hot shower. After an hour, the dose is repeated and an enema is given. The dose is repeated a third time one hour later and another hot shower enjoyed. Labor will begin 3-5 hours after the last dose if all is well.

2oz. Castor oil
2oz. vodka
2oz. orange juice
Repeat up to
three times.

★ **Blue Cohosh tincture,** 3-8 drops in a glass of warm water or tea, is very effective in starting labor. Repeat every half-hour for several hours until contractions are regular. If labor is not underway in four hours, use a dropperful of the tincture under the tongue every hour for up to four more hours or until contractions are strong and consistent.

★ Homemade or commercial herbal labor tinctures, based on Blue Cohosh and supporting herbs, are commonly used as a safe and reliable way to initiate labor. Follow the directions on the tincture bottle or take 10 drops every hour until contractions begin. One midwife uses labor tincture hourly and homeopathic Caulophyllum 200x every half-hour. She says this establishes a smooth labor within five hours. Contractions build slowly when a labor tincture is used; do not discontinue until they become regular. See Appendix II - Labor Tincture.

Problems During Labor

Stalled Labor

It is vital to determine why labor is not proceeding before using any remedies other than relaxation; oxytocic herbs are strong enough to harm the fetus or mother if there is *pelvic disparity* or other obstruction to the birth. The remedies are arranged in order of increasing strength.

Relaxation

• Tension and fear can slow and halt contractions. Support from loved ones, breath-by-breath instruction in breathing techniques, knowledge of the stages of labor, freedom to change position frequently and walk around, massage, meditation, music, and assistance (not insistence) from the birth attendants, facilitate strong contractions, normal labor, and speedy delivery.

• Five or more **calcium lactate** pills, taken once or twice, aid relaxation and encourage normal labor. So does warm milk.

• A glass of wine or beer and **jovial company** promotes relaxation and the resumption of contractions.

• To be read aloud, slowly . . .

Allow yourself to be as comfortable as possible. Feel each place where your body touches the bed (chair, floor). Around you now is a circle of protection. Only influences which are beneficial may enter here. Call your spirit guides to be with you. You share their patience, their wisdom, their strength.

Focus on your breath. Let the breath flow out of your toes and tell the toes to relax. Breathe up to the ankles, then let the breath flow out from your ankles, washing away tension. Feel the breath fill your calves and flow out as they relax. Breathe in and out of your knees. Relax the muscles and bones of your thighs as you inhale and exhale. Relax the tops of your thighs, the outsides of your thighs, the bottoms of your thighs, the inner parts of your thighs. Take the breath fully into your hip joints and let them soften and relax as the breath swirls out. Feel the entire right leg, from thigh to toes, supported by the force of gravity, held in the warm embrace of the earth. Tell the right leg to completely let go. Feel the deep relaxation of the left leg, from hip joint to foot. Give your leg to the caress of gravity. Tell both legs: "I love you. I honor you." Think about all that your legs do for you. Tell them: "You can totally relax now. I demand nothing of you."

Breathe out through your fingertips and allow them to become sensitive. Let the breath travel through your hands and ease them. Breathe into your wrists. Let your exhalation dissolve their tension. Feel the breath pass into your lower arms and tell them: "Relax." Let your elbows and upper arms relax as you breathe out. Then the shoulders, breathe through your shoulders several times until they feel free of burdens and responsibilities. Open to the release in the length of your entire right arm, shoulder to fingertips. Breathe through the whole arm. Sense your left arm and tell it once more to relax as you breathe. Let your left arm be as relaxed as your left leg and your right arm as relaxed as your right leg. Thank your arms and stroke them with your loving attention. Give them up to gravity. Let them go now.

Breathe out through your pelvis and your belly. Let your intestines relax with each breath. Breathe out of your bladder and tell it to relax. Breathe out through your uterus and let any tension flow away with your breath. (Don't be afraid to let your uterus relax; contractions don't arise from stiffness.) Give up the weight of your uterus to gravity. Feel the movement of the breath in your uterus: a smooth and rhythmic pulse. Breathe in bright and easy and breathe out soft and deep. Let go completely and feel the support of the earth beneath you.

Breathe out and relax your kidneys and the adrenal glands with them. Relax your stomach. Breathe out through your liver on the right side. Breathe out through your spleen and the pancreas on the left side. Feel the breath in your chest, and let your lungs be easy. Let your heart be easy. Feel the muscles and bones in your body and the organs lightly and safely held inside. Letting the breath come easily, breathe into and out of each vertebra. Feel the nerves settle softly in their grooves. Relax all the muscles in the back.

Breathe into your jaw and totally relax it as you breathe out. Let the muscles surrounding your lips relax. Breathe easily. Relax your ears and your cheeks as you breathe. Let the muscles around the eyes completely relax. Breathe out through the eyes. Thank your eyes and your mouth, your ears and nose for delighting you and protecting you. Let your face melt. No one is looking. No one will see. Let it all go to the mothering touch of gravity. The forehead and the scalp, even the hair, let it all go, let it all relax. Let yourself open. Let yourself be whole.

Remedies for Stalled Labor

• Finger pressure, acupuncture needling, or indirect moxa on Bladder 67 is a technique used by oriental midwives to unstall labor, augment contractions, and open and spread the pelvis. See page 57.

Also:
GOLDEN SENECIO,
FALSE VALERIAN,
COCASH WEED,
FEMALE REGULATOR,
RAGWORT, UNCUM,
COUGH WEED,
GOLDEN GROUNDSEL,
BUTTERWEED,
SWAMP SQUAWEED,
WAXWEED

• *Senecio aureus* earned its common name, **Life Root,** by speeding childbirth and helping re-establish stopped labor. The tincture of the fresh plant in flower is the most successful preparation. The usual dose of 10-15 drops in warm water may be repeated several times at half-hour intervals.

• **Labor tincture** - See Appendix II. One dose of 10-15 drops under the tongue is usually sufficient to restart a stalled labor.

★Bethroot   Widely used for birthing problems by American Indians, who preferred the white-flowered *Trillium* species, Birthroot starts and strengthens uterine contractions. One pregnant midwife reports chewing the raw root to start her labor and having immediate contractions. She also noted the acrid taste, profuse salivation, and watering of her eyes. If the tincture is used, ¼-½ teaspoon is the standard dose. You may repeat the dose twice, at thirty minute intervals, if necessary.

Oxytocic Herbs for Stalled Labor

• Marijuana leaf   *Cannabis sativa* is particularly useful if tension or emotional stress stalls the labor. It can help relax the controlling mind and bring attention to the needs of the body, as well as strengthen the needed contractions. All forms of the herb are effective, but vary tremendously in potency and dosage. Smoking offers the most control over dosage, as the effects are fairly immediate and dissipate within an hour or two. Cannabis tincture, 10 drops under the tongue, is also quick acting and the dosage can be increased slowly as desired. The greatest danger of overdose accompanies use of Cannabis tea, as the effects are slow and cumulative and several hours may pass before the full strength of the dose can be gauged. Too large a dose can cause lethargy, hallucinations, and trance-like states.

★ **Blue Cohosh root**   A strong favorite among lay midwives, *Caulophyllum thalictroides* is a reliable remedy when labor needs promoting. It does not stimulate the uterus into irregular contractions or cause any tightness or clamping down of the cervix. The usual dose is 10-20 drops of the tincture in a small glass of water, repeated hourly or as needed. The water-based infusion is not as useful as some of the active ingredients are not water-soluble. If you must rely on the infusion, try it as an enema. Many midwives use a combination of Blue and Black Cohoshes to strengthen or restart contractions. They seem to work better together than alone, a synergistic pair producing regular and coordinated contractions. NOTE: If fetal heart-tones are monitored, there may be a noticeable elevation as the Blue Cohosh starts to work. Also remember that Blue Cohosh tends to lower blood pressure.

Russian:
STEBELIST MOSHNY

Also:
BLUE GINSENG,
PAPOOSE ROOT

• **Cotton root bark**   The herb of choice in areas where cotton is grown, *Gossypium* root bark infusion is taken in sips to induce strong uterine contractions. Cotton root bark is highly recommended for prolonged labors where the mother is very tired, and for labors that start and stop.

Rigid Os

The softening cervix may stay rigid at the opening, or os, impeding dilation and slowing labor. If the os feels hard, stiff, or elastic to the touch use these remedies combined or as simples.

• Take a hot bath; relax; **open** to your labor; listen to music.

• Change your environment completely. If you are inside, go out for a walk. If you can't go out, move to a different room.

• **Oil of Evening Primrose** rubbed directly on the cervix encourages softening and opening. Squeeze the oil out of several capsules onto your fingers. Rub your fingers slowly around and into the os, holding the os open through two or three contractions.

• One midwife uses sips of **Spikenard** root infusion (*Aralia racemosa* or *A. nudicaulis*) to relax a hard cervix.

• Ten drops of **Labor tincture** under the tongue or in some water is usually effective in relaxing the os.

★ **Lobelia tincture** is recommended by virtually every herbalist and midwife for rigid os uteri with rigid rim, *perineal* and vaginal rigidity in labor. *Lobelia inflata* can relax every voluntary muscle in the body if given in a large enough dose; an insufficient dose is stimulating. The effect is transitory, rarely lasting more than thirty minutes, and sometimes less than fifteen. Use 60-150 drops of the tincture of fresh Lobelia leaf, flower, and seed, in a quarter glass of water. The dose may be repeated two times, at thirty minute intervals, or until the os relaxes.

If you are unsure of the strength and effect of the tincture you are using, experiment with it. A sufficiently large dose will usually cause some strange sensations such as tingling in the extremities, flushing, and a rubbery feeling in the face. Smaller doses will increase nervous energy, encourage talkativeness, and lighten the mood. CAUTION: Lobelia is considered a dangerous herb. It may produce nausea, stupor, intense burning in the throat, and other individual side effects.

Exhaustion

These remedies safely increase energy during childbirth.

★ Ginger root   Teas and tinctures of (cultivated) *Zingiber* and Wild Ginger, *Asarum canadense*, bring energy to the pelvis.

Cultivated Ginger increases the chi (life energy) and aids mental focus. Use it fresh, dried, or powdered. In each cup of water, steep one ounce of the grated fresh root, one quarter ounce of the shredded dried root, *or* one half to one teaspoonful of the powder, for 5-30 minutes. Sip the tea throughout labor to maintain energy. To increase energy, use a full cup as often as every thirty minutes, or try 15-20 drops of the tincture in a cup of water or Raspberry leaf infusion.

Wild Ginger increases the energy of the *root chakra*

and reduces mental resistance to the birthing process. The tea, made by brewing a teaspoonful of dried roots (actually rhizomes) in a cup of water for 5-15 minutes, can be sipped when needed or throughout the birth. The tincture draws energy more rapidly; use 2-5 drops under the tongue; repeat no more than three times.

CAUTION: Ginger increases circulation to the uterus and may increase risk of hemorrhage postpartum if used within an hour of the birth.

• Ginseng root   Though primarily used to gradually build energy, *Panax quinquefolius* and *P. schinseng* can lend enough immediate energy to a difficult labor to make a difference. The traditional method is to chew on a piece of Seng during the entire labor. If you can't manage that, capsules, extracts, and liquid preparations of Ginseng are a good second choice for this application. Avoid teas, which are made from the less effective tails; avoid powders which combine Ginseng with vitamin C, its natural antagonist; avoid tablets or capsules which combine other herbs with the Ginseng. Dosage is dependent on the form and strength of the Ginseng preparation being used. A usual dose of capsules is 2-4 (eight grain) every four hours up to six times.

Also:
DIVINE HERB,
WONDER ROOT,
FLOWER OF LIFE,
SEED OF EARTH,
SANTA ROOT,
IMMORTALITY ROOT,
PANACEA

• A slow warm **molasses enema** can dramatically increase energy. Use 1-2 tablespoons molasses well dissolved in a quart of water. Ten drops of Ginger or Ginseng tincture may be included if desired.

Pain

I was talking with a friend recently who fumed that no one had told her that having a baby would hurt. She was in labor for 36 hours and begging for anything to ease the pain. For me, it was easier, but my back hurt. Each one of us experiences the sensation and energy of our childbirth differently, but we all agree some parts of it are ouch. All of these herbal pain relievers work better with the pain meditations in *Who Dies*. (The meditations also work alone.)

• **Motherwort** tincture produces a floating or non-existent feeling in the uterus; not so good if labor is irregular, but just right for the early achey part of a regular labor when the actual birth is still hours away. Use five drops in a glass of water. The effect is noticeable within twenty minutes and gradually fades over 1-3 hours. Repeat as needed.

• **Skullcap** tincture is my favorite remedy for pain of all kinds. Simple pain, such as headache or the strong sensation accompanying the dilation of the cervix, usually responds to a single dose of 3-8 drops Skullcap. You can repeat the dose whenever necessary, but watch out for its sedative effect.

• Use 25-30 drops of tincture of fresh **St. Joan's Wort** to control spasms in the back, sides, and uterus.

• Skullcap and St. Joan's Wort complement each other wonderfully. A combined dose of 3 drops Skullcap and 25 drops St. Joan's Wort can be used as often as every hour, or as needed, to ease pain.

Elevated Blood Pressure

Hypertension during labor can be a problem; these herbal remedies are safe and effective.

• **Relax** deeply, and strongly visualize open blood vessels. For a stronger effect, combine with 10 drops of Skullcap, Valerian, or **Passionflower** tincture.

• Fresh Garlic or Garlic oil capsules can lower blood pressure. Eat several large raw cloves or take up to 15 capsules.

• Steep a handful each of dried **Hops, Skullcap,** and **Valerian** in a quart of water for at least two hours and drink a cupful. The effect lasts one or two hours. Repeat the dose as necessary or sip the brew throughout labor to maintain consistent blood pressure readings. The taste of this brew is remarkably acrid, bitter, and strong.

• Use 10-20 drops each of Skullcap and Valerian tinctures in a cup of warm water or herbal tea. This dose gradually diminishes in effectiveness over a period of several hours. To sustain the effect, use the tinctures in Hops tea and sip slowly, or repeat the dose. This preparation is a little better tasting than the previous one.

Problems After the Birth

Expulsion of the Placenta

The final contractions of labor cause the placenta to separate from the uterus and be expelled, usually within thirty minutes of the baby's birth. If the uterus is atonic and does not contract well, this normal process may not occur or may occur only partially. The three variations of this process are: 1) the placenta is totally adhered (still attached to the uterine wall); 2) the placenta is partially adhered, partially detached; 3) the placenta is completely detached, but still retained in the uterus. The first two possibilities are likely to be combined with active bleeding. Management of this stage of labor usually calls for getting the placenta out before dealing with hemorrhage, so time can be an important consideration here. These remedies are listed in order of increasing strength.

Retained Placenta, Normal Bleeding

• Use **Raspberry leaf** infusion to help facilitate placenta delivery. Chips of frozen Raspberry leaf infusion sucked throughout the labor help keep the uterus working strongly and smoothly.

• If the uterus is contracting, but not strongly, and the delivery of the placenta is slow, try squatting, pushing with the contractions, massaging the uterus, and stimulating the nipples, either by manipulation or sucking.

German:
GUNDLEREBE,
GUNDERMANN

French:
LIERRE TERRESTRE

Also:
GILL-OVER-THE-
GROUND, CAT'S
FOOT, CREEPING
JENNY, ALE HOOF,
HAY MAIDS

Spanish:
ANGELICA

German:
ENGELWURZ

French:
ANGELINE

Also:
MASTERWORT,
PURPLE ANGELICA,
ALEXANDERS,
ARCHANGEL

★ Ground Ivy herb

Glechoma hederacea is an old specific for bringing down the placenta. I first used Ground Ivy by feeding the fresh plant to kidding goats to insure expulsion of the afterbirth. Midwives in the mountains offer a cupful of the infusion of **Ground Ivy, Catnip,** or **Basil** leaves immediately after the birth and say they never have a retained afterbirth. If Ground Ivy tincture is available, ½-1 teaspoonful is used as a dose.

★ Angelicas

The archangel roots are powerful emmenagogues and uterine stimulants, highly recommended for dealing with a fully adhered placenta. *Angelica archangelica, A. sylvestris, A. atropurpurea,* and *A. sinensis* (Dong Quai) are used by midwives around the world. A single 30-50 drop dose of the root tincture under the tongue usually works in five minutes. If contractions don't resume within fifteen minutes, repeat the dose. Angelica root syrup is traditional among some midwives who use a tablespoonful dose and say the placenta arrives ten minutes later. CAUTION: Some women are quite sensitive to substances in Angelica. Fresh root tinctures may cause more reactions than dried root preparations. John Lust claims "untoward effects on blood pressure, heart action, and respiration" with large doses of A. archangelica, but I have no verification of this.

Undelivered Placenta, Heavy Bleeding

★ American Mistletoe leaf

An infusion of *Phoradendron* leaves finds favor with midwives who brew it at the beginning of labor and use it at the end to quiet the nerves, stimulate uterine contractions, expel the placenta, and stop hemorrhage. The leaves are tough and alkaloid-rich, so use an ounce in a pint of boiling water and steep for at least eight hours. The usual dose is ¼ cup, which may be repeated as the situation demands. CAUTION: Mistletoe berries are considered deadly poisonous. The alkaloids in Mistletoe leaves and berries stimulate the heart and central nervous system, raise blood pressure, and contract the uterine smooth muscle.

• Put 50 drops of Ground Ivy or **Angelica** tincture **and** 20 drops **Blue Cohosh** or Labor tincture under the tongue to cause rapid emptying and clamping down of the uterus. Repeat in 2-5 minutes if necessary.

• Witch Hazel bark   The tincture of fresh or dried *Hamamelis* bark stops bleeding rapidly through its powerful *hemostatic* and astringent actions, and does not constrict the os or slow down the emergence of the afterbirth. Ten to twenty drops of **Witch Hazel tincture** under the tongue can be used repeatedly to control bleeding until the placenta is delivered. Note: Witch Hazel does not help expel the placenta.

Spanish:
HOJAS DE HAMAMELIS

German:
VIRGINISCHER
ZAUBERSTRAUCH

French:
NOISETIER DES
SORCIÈRES

Also:
WINTER BLOOM,
SPOTTED ALDER,
SNAPPING HAZEL

Hemorrhage

Blood loss during childbirth is called hemorrhage if it exceeds two cups. The hemorrhage may be a prolonged, slow seeping or a dramatic sudden gushing. Ninety percent of maternal hemorrhages occur because the uterus, lacking muscle tone, remains large and flabby, and does not clamp down and restrict the flow of blood. Hemorrhage is also caused by insufficient vitamin K in the blood and the resultant slow clotting, a placenta which tears away or separates partially from the uterus, a precipitous delivery, an especially large baby, and tearing of vaginal or cervical tissue. Low hemoglobin is not a direct factor in postpartum hemorrhage, but is of concern as it increases the risk of complications if hemorrhage does occur. Massive hemorrhage is usually obvious; the slower seeping hemorrhage is more dangerous as it can be overlooked in the excitement surrounding the newborn infant. These remedies, increasing in strength from first to last, are useful in many situations.

Hemorrhage Prevention

★ **Nettle** or **Alfalfa leaf infusion** or tea taken throughout the pregnancy will increase available vitamin K and hemoglobin in the blood. Several cups of infusion consumed throughout the labor will have a less pronounced but beneficial preventative action.

• Midwives who give 10 drops of **Motherwort** tincture to every mother after the baby is born claim that it totally prevents hemorrhage. The "little mother" is soothing and calming and a fine uterine tonic.

• **Shepherd's Purse** is useful as a hemorrhage remedy but not as prevention. One midwife gave several dropperful doses of fresh Shepherd's Purse tincture to several women during labor to prevent postpartum hemorrhage and found that it encouraged the formation of huge blood clots. These clots were painfully hard to pass and sometimes kept the uterus from clamping down.

Remedies for Postpartum Hemorrhage

• **Witch Hazel** bark tincture, 20 drops under the tongue, is used when hemorrhage occurs before the afterbirth is delivered. See page 71.

★ Lady's Mantle   The charming European plant, *Alchemilla vulgaris,* is renowned for its ability to cure all manner of "female problems" but is difficult to find or buy in America. It grows fairly easily and can be harvested and tinctured after two years. The tincture of the fresh root is an excellent blood coagulant in doses of 20-30 drops, repeated as necessary.

• Tinctures of oxytocic herbs such as Blue Cohosh, Cotton root bark, or Cannabis, used in combination with a hemostatic herb such as Witch Hazel or Lady's Mantle, slow a hemorrhage caused by uterine atony. The usual dose is 10 drops oxytocic herb tincture and 20 drops hemostatic herb tincture, under the tongue, repeated as necessary.

• **Cayenne caution:** Although *Capsicum* is recommended by some herbalists as successful in controlling postpartum bleeding, this fast-acting herb is in disfavor among midwives; some go so far as to call it dangerous. It does slow down a hemorrhage, but it also stimulates circulation. The danger hides in a false sense of security: having seemingly alleviated the problem, the midwife tends to other concerns, only to find that the hemorrhage has returned with increased vigor behind her back. In addition, Cayenne does not contract the uterus, a necessity if bleeding is to be totally controlled.

★ Shepherd's Purse herb   The common weed, *Capsella bursa-pastoris,* is an amazing blood coagulant and *vasoconstrictor* with a special affinity for women. The tincture of the fresh plant in flower not only stops bleeding, but also promotes uterine contractions, making it a specific simple for postpartum hemorrhage. The dried herb loses its power rapidly, so infusions and tinctures of the dried plant (most commercial tinctures and so-called extracts are made from dried plant material) are not optimally effective. Be certain of the action of your Shepherd's Purse tincture by making it yourself from fresh plants in the spring or by buying it from an herbalist who prepares the tinctures from fresh plants. A dropperful of the fresh plant tincture (20-40 drops) under the tongue can stop postpartum hemorrhage in five seconds! Thirty seconds is the longest any midwife has reported it taking to significantly slow or completely stop bleeding. If you are forced to use a tincture or extract of dried plants, try one teaspoonful (150 drops) under the tongue, and repeat every minute or as needed.

German:
HIRTENTÄSCHELKRAUT,
TÄSCHENKRAUT

French:
BOURSE-À-PASTEUR,
CAPSELLE

Chinese: CHI-TS'AI

Russian:
PASTUSHYA SUMKA

Also:
MOTHER'S HEART,
PICKOOCKER, CASE-
WORT, SHEPHERD'S
SPROUT, SHOVEL
WEED, SHEPHERD'S
BAG

• Postpartum Hemorrhage Formulae - See Appendix II

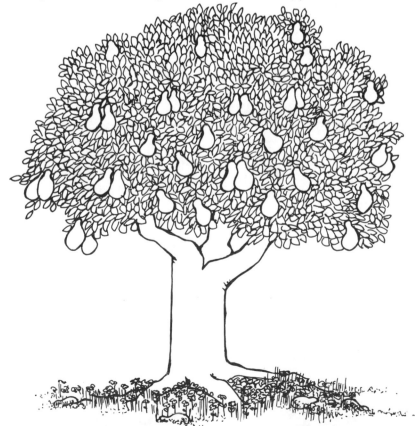

Shock

Large blood loss may lead to *shock*. Even when the blood loss is not dramatic, blood pressure may drop dangerously. Be alert to any faintness, dizziness, nausea, thirst, weakness, pallor, or restlessness in the mother. These remedies are adequate for shockiness, but not for clinical shock which is life threatening and demands immediate attention. If the blood pressure, pulse, and respirations are unstable, and the pupils of the eyes are dilated, seek emergency help without delay.

• A woman feeling shocky or in shock must stay awake and must lay down with her legs well elevated or wrapped from the ankle up in ace bandages to help keep blood supply to the vital organs adequate. She will be chilly; keep her warm. She may be nervous; reassure her. She may be restless; keep her still. She may want to sleep; keep her awake and talking.

• A few drops of Bach **Rescue Remedy** under the tongue is a trusted remedy for shockiness. It's good for calming midwives, too! The dose may be repeated every five minutes for as long as needed.

• Homeopathic **Arnica 30x** given every five minutes is said to stabilize and reverse beginning shock.

• **Motherwort** tincture acts quickly to calm the feelings, strengthen the heart, and allay shockiness. The usual dose is 10 drops under the tongue, once. CAUTION: Bleeding may be increased by use of repeated doses.

• **Lobelia** tincture in small and repeated doses is specific for shock. Use 3-5 drops under the tongue, repeated every five minutes as required.

• A mixture of one teaspoon **table salt** and a half teaspoon **baking soda** dissolved in four cups of warm water and drunk freely can help keep the *electrolyte* balance stable and forestall clinical shock. CAUTION: Give nothing by mouth unless the person is fully conscious.

References & Resources

- *Herbs for Women: A Guide for Lay Midwives*
  Valerie Hobbs; 1980, Informed Homebirth
  POB 3675, Ann Arbor, MI 48106

- *Nature's Healing Agents*
  R. Swinburne Clymer, MD; 1905, Dorrance & Co.

- *Spiritual Midwifery*
  Ina May Gaskin; 1978, The Book Publishing Co.

- *Guide to Midwifery*
  Elizabeth Davis; 1981, John Muir Publications

- *Who Dies*
  Stephen Levine; 1982, Doubleday

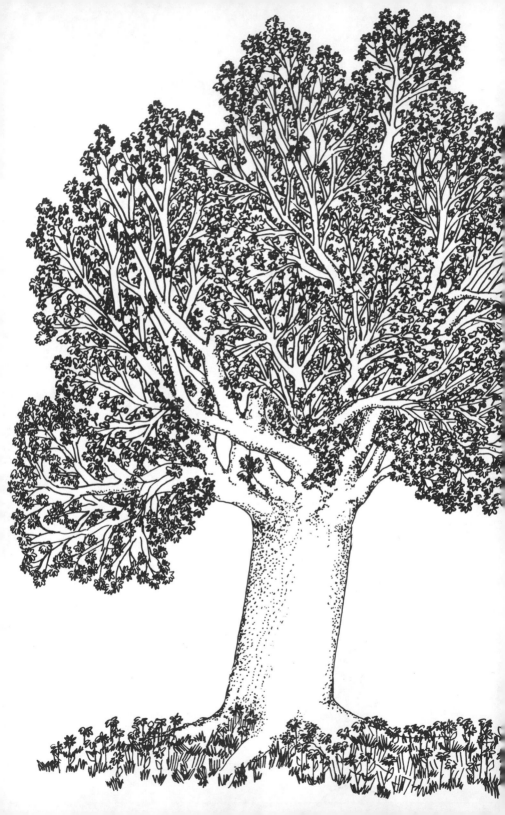

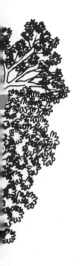

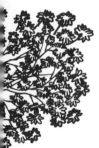

After Pregnancy

The first days after the birth encompass great transitions. Your uterus shrinks rapidly, your breasts engorge and lactation commences, your vagina heals from the stretching or tearing of birth, your liver and kidneys process a sudden and large influx of hormones, and you adjust to a new sleep pattern. You feel intensely and variously, full of fear, resistant to change, depressed, ecstatic, erotic. You experience the inner movements of separation and bonding, diminishment and fulfillment. When all flows easily, Wise Woman herbs assist and encourage the shrinking, the lactating, the healing, the processing, the adjusting, the feeling, and the centering. If there are difficulties, Wise Woman herbs help the repairing, the replacing, and the resistance to bacteria and yeasts. To the best of my knowledge, all the herbs in this section are safe for use by nursing mothers.

Perineal Tears

The *perineum* must stretch far beyond its ordinary limits as the infant emerges. Many women's bodies are capable of this, but some are not and the skin gives way and tears. "Just in case she tears" an *episiotomy* is a standard pre-birth procedure in most hospitals. I was told that if I refused to have an episiotomy my vagina would be ripped to shreds and I would never enjoy sex again. I have heard that this cutting was instituted for the maintenance of men's sexual pleasure; in some parts of Africa, the vaginal opening is sewn tight to increase male pleasure and must be cut open at the birth of each child! If the perineum fails to stretch enough to allow the head to be born, a cut can easily be made (without the use of anesthetics) while the crown is against the perineum; there is seldom a need to cut beforehand. A cut is considered preferable to a tear by the medical profession, as it is easier to *suture*, but most women and midwives prefer tears. One midwife puts it this way: "Tears (although possibly ragged and therefore needing more skill to sew) heal easier and quicker, usually involve less depth and tissue damage, are less painful, and heal with less scar tissue." Another midwife says that she has found that many tears do not need suturing since they *approximate* well and that they heal better without stitches. The following remedies can be used equally well for healing minor tears, lacerations, or surgical cuts.

King Louis XIV liked to see his mistresses give birth, so he instituted a new position giving him a better view: flat on the back.

Preventing Perineal Tears

• **Massage,** soften, and stretch the perineum throughout the pregnancy with the aid of olive oil, Comfrey ointment, wheat germ oil, lanolin, or sesame oil.

• Use warmed oil or hot **compresses** of herbs such as Plantain or Comfrey leaves during labor to encourage pliability of the perineum.

• Try a **birthing position** that puts different pressure on the perineum. Hands and knees, squatting, and semi-sitting are much less likely to provoke tears than lying flat on the back.

• Use **controlled breathing** to avoid rapid emergence as the head crowns and slides down the vaginal canal.

Remedies for Perineal Tears

★ Comfrey leaf   Drink it and sit in it! Drinking a cup a day of *Symphytum* leaf infusion builds new cells rapidly and helps alleviate pain. A sitz bath soothes and heals, keeps the tissues flexible, and holds itching to a minimum.

German:
SCHWARZWURZ,
BEIN WELL

French:
GRANDE CONSOUDE

Russian:
OKOPNIK

• Herbal **sitz baths** help prevent infection, aid healing, and offer pain relief. Yarrow, Rosemary, Golden Seal, Oak bark, Witch Hazel, Sea Grape bark, Myrrh and many others are useful. See page 32 for sitz bath instructions. CAUTION: If you have stitches, limit sitz baths to one a day.

★ Aloe Vera gel   Bottled Aloe Vera often contains preservatives which irritate sensitive skin, so—though it is a bit more work—use the gel from the fresh plant to make a poultice to heal and cool a torn perineum. Remove the green skin from several leaves, place the clear gel on a gauze pad or menstrual pad, hold or tape it in place. Aloe is remarkably pain killing when applied this way. Replace the poultice with a fresh one when the pain returns.

• Slippery Elm bark   A paste of *Ulmus fulva* powder, water, and olive oil or vitamin E oil, used directly on the tear or incision, binds together torn tissue, soothes pain, and strengthens the skin surface. Comfrey root powder added to this paste speeds the healing.

• Well known for its ability to promote scar-free healing, **vitamin E** is best used after the tear is well closed, or after the third day on a sutured wound. Frequent applications are most effective. Take special care with cleanliness, as the oil attracts dirt, *lochia*, etc. and could promote infection. Also be sure to use only pure vitamin E oil, as synthetics and preparations often contain flavoring oils and substances not intended for use on sensitive skin surfaces.

• Note to Midwives: A dropperful of Valerian tincture under the mother's tongue stops shakes so you can suture neatly.

After-pains

The baby is born, the placenta expelled, now the uterus continues to contract as it returns to its normal, non-pregnant, size. If you have had two or more births, you may experience intense pain (sometimes worse than labor pains) with these after-birth contractions, but it is very unusual to have after-pains with the first birth. Your favorite menstrual cramp reliever can be used for after-pains, or try these remedies, which are arranged in order of increasing strength.

Preventing After-pains

• There is a strong possibility that a daily dose of 5 drops of **Liferoot** (*Senecio aureus*) tincture in water for two to four weeks preceeding the birth will prevent after-pains. It relieves even the worst menstrual cramping if taken daily for two weeks before the flow.

• **Rest** in bed for several days after the birth and make frequent trips to empty your bladder. This regime keeps the uterus firm and low, which helps prevent bloodclots and pooling blood—both of which increase after-pains.

• The rhythmic **sucking** of your newly born child, even before the milk comes in, is soothing and reassuring to both of you, and helps your uterus to contract smoothly and quickly. This lessens the duration of the after-pains, but increases the intensity.

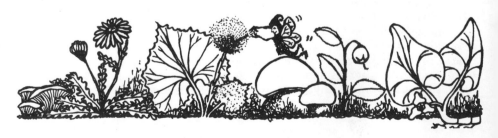

Remedies for After-pains

• One or two cups daily of **Ground Ivy** leaf infusion eases after-pains and promotes good uterine tone.

• Catnip leaves   Well known as a menstrual cramp brew, *Nepeta cataria* is right at home in dealing with after-pains. It relieves spasms of the uterus, keeps the after-flow moving out easily and clot free, relaxes nervous tension, and acts as a very effective pain killer. Several different preparations are effective: tea, tincture, or cigarettes. The tea is quite pleasant and may be drunk freely. The effect of Catnip tincture is cumulative; second and subsequent doses may make you sleepy or non-functional; 10-30 drops is the usual dose. Catnip cigarettes act quickly if you inhale deeply.

• After-pain Brew - See Appendix II

★ Motherwort herb   In addition to relieving after-pains, *Leonurus cardiaca* helps tone the uterus and ease the nervous system. Preparation and dosage is quite variable; I use the tincture exclusively, but some prefer the tea. Many women respond strongly to 5 drops of tincture in a glass of water, others require 20 drops before noticing any effect. One cup of tea is all that is tolerable as the taste is quite bitter. "Perhaps," one woman surmises, "you decide the cramps aren't so bad after you taste that brew!"

German:
HERZGESPANN

French:
AGRIPAUME
    CARDIAQUE

Chinese:
TSAN · TS'AI

Russian:
PUSTIRNIK
    SERDECHNY

Also:
HEART HERB,
LION'S EAR/TAIL

Child-bed Fever

Midwives of every era have understood the need for cleanliness during the birthing when infection can readily enter the bloodstream through the open os and uterus. Postpartum infections increased dramatically with the intervention of obstetrics. My maternal grandmother had her first four children (including twins) safely at home. Pressured into having her fifth, my mother, in a hospital, she died within a week of the birth—from child-bed fever. If she had known about these Wise Woman remedies, I might have known her.

★ Echinacea root   The herbalists' antibiotic is *Echinacea augustifolia,* also known as Purple Coneflower or Kansas Snake Root. I have seen it clear up serious cases of blood poisoning, mastitis, strep and staph infections, pneumonia, and other systemic infections. Unlike penicillin, it works as a preventative as well as a curative. If child-bed fever seems likely for any reason (clean conditions were impossible to maintain, you are severely run-down or malnourished, etc.), a week's course of Echinacea will decrease the possibility of infection. If infection is present, use the Echinacea for at least a week, but expect response (diminishment of fever) within 48 hours.

• As a **preventative:** use 10-15 drops of Echinacea tincture in a glass of water twice a day for a minimum of five days.

• As a **curative:** use two cups of Echinacea infusion daily for five days, then one cup of infusion daily for another five days. It is important to continue the Echinacea for the full ten days, even though the fever will abate within three to five days and the cure will seem to be complete within a week. If only tincture is available, use ½ drop per pound of body weight as the measure of a dose. Repeat the dose three or four times a day until the fever abates, then two times a day for another week.

• Fever Brew   Echinacea is an excellent fever herb, but you may also wish to use an infusion of Yarrow and Peppermint to sweat the fever out. Prepare an infusion using one ounce of each of the two herbs in a half gallon jar. Begin drinking in two hours, while still hot. Leave the herbs to steep in the water as you continue to drink the brew. CAUTION: Do not use if you are in a weak condition. Do not use Yarrow alone if your fever is over 102°; it may temporarily increase the fever.

Depression

Postpartum depression is related to the rapid readjustment of hormones in the mother's body after the birth. Herbs which aid the body in rebalancing hormones are given here, along with other remedies.

• Figs, sprouts, royal jelly, bee pollen, Ginseng, Hops, and Sarsaparilla help the body process and balance hormones.

• **Breast feeding** is probably the best cure for postpartum depression. The process helps moderate hormonal swings, increases the *endorphin* level and allows your body to regain hormonal balance slowly and evenly.

• Lemon Balm leaves   Considered a specific for helping one cope with life situations that are difficult to accept, such as the many unexpected changes a new child brings to its parents, *Melissa* is an old favorite for depression, melancholy, and hysteria. One or two cups of the good tasting infusion, mellowed with milk and honey, every day for a week or two will suffice.

★ Blessed Thistle leaves   The intensely bitter Milk Thistle has a wide reputation for alleviating many postpartum problems, including severe depression. Use a cup or two of the infusion daily, or up to 80 drops per day of the equally effective, but not so bitter, tincture.

• Postpartum Depression Brew - See Appendix II

Exhaustion/Tension

The energy of childbirth is a great high and many women don't need or want to sleep right afterwards, but sometimes the energy load becomes an overload. Exhaustion after a normal birth, even a prolonged one, is easily resolved by providing the mother with quiet time for a nap. But exhaustion combined with tension—worry about the newborn, the aftermath of a painful and difficult labor, the sense of failure if the planned delivery had to be changed or compromised, and so on—can prevent sleep. These remedies are safe and sure ways to induce calmness and sleep. Try them in the order listed, mildest first. The best herb for the job is the softest one that works.

• Chamomile flowers   The popularity of German or Garden Chamomile testifies to its potency as a calming sleep inducer, pain-killer, and mental relaxer. Brew the flowers briefly, a teaspoon to a cup of water, and drink the pleasantly aromatic tea freely. Several cups of hot tea with milk and honey may be necessary to induce sleep.

● **Motherwort herb**   Clear-minded, non-drowsy relief from the tension and confusion of overwhelming emotion is the promise of Motherwort tincture. Use 5 drops in a glass of water, repeated as needed. CAUTION: Excessive use of Motherwort tincture (more than four doses a day for several weeks) may cause you to become dependent on it.

Also:
MAD·DOG WEED,
BLUE PIMPERNEL,
HELMET FLOWER,
HOOD·WORT,
SIDE·FLOWER,
HOODED WILLOW
HERB, MAD WEED

★ **Skullcap herb**   The tincture, not the infusion, of *Scutellaria lateriflora* sedates and brings on sound sleep. A friend who could not sleep without the aid of Seconal reported that only 3 drops of (homemade) Skullcap tincture put him immediately to sleep. Another friend took 5 drops of tincture to calm down and didn't awaken until sixteen hours later! There are no side effects from overdoses of Skullcap, so start small but don't be afraid to repeat or increase the dose, especially when using commercial tinctures made from dried Skullcap. Skullcap tincture is not habit forming.

● **Hops flowers**   *Humulus lupulus* is a strong seducer of sleep. I have seen insomniacs slumped on the kitchen table with half a cup of Hops infusion still beside them! Hops is also an excellent herb for increasing and enriching breast milk. It is also helpful in relieving after-pains. Unfortunately, the taste of Hops is acrid and unpalatable to many and the tincture does not seem to be as effective.

Lactation

Galactagogues

Of the many herbs and foods used to encourage and increase the milk flow, these are perennial favorites of midwives, mothers, and Wise Women.

• Simple teas or infusions of **nourishing herbs** such as Comfrey, Raspberry leaf, Nettles, Alfalfa, or Red Clover encourage a plentiful supply of breast milk and a relaxed, healthy mother. These mineral rich nourishing herbs also protect you from mineral loss during the stress of nursing and infant care. Rotate, using each one for a week, to derive the unique benefits that each offers.

• Apricots, asparagus, green beans, carrots, sweet potatoes, peas, pecans, and all **leafy greens** such as beet greens, Parsley, Watercress, and Dandelion leaves are considered helpful in increasing and sustaining lactation.

• Blessed Thistle leaves   Famed for its ability to increase milk supply, *Cnicus benedictus* is best used as a tincture; up to 20 drops, two to four times daily is the usual dose. It is said to remove suicidal feelings and lift depression as well. It used to be called Our Lady's Milk Thistle. Rarely found on the east coast, Blessed Thistle is a weed in almost every west coast garden I've visited.

• Borage leaves   *Borago officinalis* acts like a weed in the garden, spreading its large leaves and lovely blue flowers over a huge area, threatening to overrun the plot, and scattering its seeds everywhere to insure more plants next year. But it is worth growing, even with the potential danger of a never-ending supply of Borage! The leaves are most highly regarded as a tea for increasing milk flow, and the flowers are a delight in salads. Half a cupful of Borage infusion at each nursing insures an abundant supply of milk, acts as a mild laxative, and soothes jangled nerves.

★ Fennel/Barley Water   Prepare barley water by soaking ½ cup pearled (regular) barley in 3 cups cold water overnight or by boiling for 25 minutes. Strain out barley and discard or add to a soup. Heat a cup or two of the barley water to boiling as needed, store the rest in the refrigerator. Pour 1 cup boiling barley water over 1 teaspoon Fennel seeds and steep for no longer than 30 minutes. This combination not only increases the breast milk, but eases after-pains and settles the digestion of mom and babe.

• **Hops flowers**   An old, old remedy for mothers of twins who need lots more milk, *Humulus* is a suitable accompaniment to nighttime feedings, as it brings sleep along with increased milk flow. Beer is a convenient source of Hops and is far tastier than tea or infusion. I vividly recall an older woman with mammoth breasts sitting down next to me in the park one day as I breast fed my daughter. "I nursed eight children, two sets of twins," she said smilingly, "all on beer!" Be aware that domestic beers contain potentially harmful chemicals. Some imported beers are additive-free. There are also alcohol- and chemical-free brews of Hops and malt available: "Moussy" from Switzerland, for example.

• Galacatagogue Brew - See Appendix II

Painful Breasts

There are three main causes of painful breasts. 1) A blocked milk tube or duct can cause swelling of the breast and acute pain. It usually feels like a bruised lump, and a red streak may radiate out from it. 2) Mastitis, an infection in the breast, causes pain also, and is generally accompanied by fever and acute tenderness and redness of the breast. The infected breast may become hard, lumpy, and swollen. 3) An oversupply of milk, or a decision not to nurse at all, engorges the breasts and usually causes some pain. The first remedies are useful for all these conditions; the latter ones are more specific.

Poultices for Sore Breasts

Poultices, compresses, and soaks are the best general first aid for painful breasts. Hot water alone has a beneficial effect, as it stimulates circulation and eases the tension in taut tissues; herbs increase the effectiveness. Frequent (4-5 times a day), short (3-5 minute), consistent applications work better than sporadic, lengthy treatments. If infection is present, throw away poulticing materials after use. If there is no infection, brews and towels may be reused a number of times.

• Run a sink full of warm water. Bend over it with your breasts in the sink. Allow the milk to flow out, massaging down from the back of the breast. This relieves engorgement and eases pain.

• Use a hot compress of **Parsley** to ease swollen and painful breasts. Place a handful of fresh or dried Parsley leaves in a clean cotton diaper, tie with a rubber band, and steep in simmering water for 10-15 minutes. Compress the breast with the hot, wet bundle.

• Try a hot compress of **Comfrey leaves,** fresh or dried, to soothe sore nipples, soften engorged tissues, reduce the pain of swollen breasts, and help unblock tubes and ducts. Prepare and use like Parsley.

• Prepare a cold poultice of grated **raw potato** to draw out the heat of inflammation, localize infection, and unblock clogged tubes. Grate raw potato and apply directly to the breasts, covering with a clean cloth. Remove or replace when dry.

• Soak breasts in slippery and slimy **Marshmallow root**. It delightfully soothes tender tissues, opens clogged ducts and tubes, powerfully draws out infection, and diminishes the pain of engorged, inflamed breasts and sore nipples. Make an infusion of the dried root, steeping two ounces in a half gallon of boiling water overnight. Reheat the infusion to near boiling. Pour it into a sink or basin and soak the breasts until the infusion cools.

• Gently warm a handful of dried Elder blossoms in just enough olive oil to cover; keep warm for twenty minutes. Strain, cool, and rub the oil into nipples and breasts to relieve pain and sensitivity.

Remedies for Blocked Tube or Duct

• Continue nursing on a breast with a blocked or plugged tube. Cessation of nursing can increase the discomfort and endanger the milk supply. But go carefully; nurse or pump every hour but just enough to empty the breast.

• Right before nursing, use any of the above warm compresses for five or ten minutes (they all taste fine).

• Be sure to get plenty of rest. The blockage will usually clear within a few hours or overnight.

Remedies for Mastitis

• Treatment of mastitis with herbs should include: 1) hot applications to the breast at least four times daily (see pages 86-87 for poultices), 2) plenty of bed rest, and 3) nursing as often and as long as possible on the infected breast.

• Breast infections are almost always a sign of too little rest. Time to take a daily nap, and ten minute breaks every two hours: put your feet up, enjoy a cup of Violet leaf infusion; relax deeply. It is important to nurse often, keeping the breasts empty to promote prompt healing. (The breast infection won't make your infant sick.)

Spanish: CONGORA

Chinese: SHANG·LU

Russian: FITALAKA AMERIKANA

Also: INKBERRY, PIGEON BERRY, CROWBERRY, COAKUM, POCAN, COCUM, CHONGRAS, COKAN, GARGET, CANCER ROOT, SKOKE, RED·INK PLANT, JALAP

★ **Poke root**   *Phytolacca*
is a widespread, noticeable weed with tall magenta stalks and black berries. A tincture of the fresh (only) root stimulates lymph gland activity and clears mastitis quickly. Poke root is potent and the effect is cumulative; use no more than 2 drops daily. I usually combine Poke with Echinacea, but it may be effective as a simple.

• **Propolis** is a substance secreted by bees as a glue. It has a history of use against infection in Russia and a strong following among midwives in North America. It is said to accelerate healing time by increasing the body's metabolism and general resistance to disease. A dose of the tincture is 10-15 drops twice a day; it combines well with Echinacea.

• Elder root, dug and grated fresh into boiling water, makes an excellent poultice for mastitis. See pages 117-118 before you use Elder.

★ Echinacea root   *Echinacea augustifolia* is an excellent treatment for even severe cases of mastitis. My most recent experience bears this out. A goat in my herd had triplets which she nursed for two weeks, until we sold two of them. The last one nursed for several months, during which time we noticed that the milk tasted a bit "off." Assuming the goat had intestinal worms, we dosed her with garlic, but the taste remained. We discovered why within a day of selling the last kid: the goat promptly ran 5 degrees of fever! She had had mastitis all the while, but without any swelling, tenderness, clots or blood in the milk. With such an entrenched case, treatment was difficult. To make it even harder, the goat refused to eat or drink for three days, during which time her temperature remained 4-5 degrees above normal. We forced Echinacea tincture down her throat three times a day until she resumed eating, then we offered her Echinacea infusion in milk and the dried root in a little bit of grain. Three to four times a day, we poulticed her udder with hot cabbage leaves. Within two weeks the mastitis was cleared.

I much prefer the action of Echinacea as an infusion. Use one ounce of the root in a pint of boiling water and steep it for at least eight hours. Drink two cups daily until the fever comes down. Then make a lighter infusion: one ounce of the root in a quart of boiling water and drink one or two cups daily for another week.

If you must resort to the tincture: use ½ drop per pound of body weight as a single dose. Repeat the dose up to six times a day until the fever remits. Continue with two to three doses daily for another seven days or until all symptoms are cleared.

Remedies for Engorgement

• Drink **Sage tea** or infusion. Sage is an anti-galactagogue and dries up the flow of milk.

• Take 2 drops of Poke root tincture daily to decrease swelling. The same dose can be used to prevent engorgement.

Caked, Sore Nipples

Although sore nipples heal rapidly, often within a day or two, it is easier to prevent them than to treat them. If your nipples are persistently or suddenly sore, you might suspect a thrush infection. Further symptoms of thrush include pink, flaky skin and itchy nipples. See pages 109-110 for thrush remedies. Neither sore nipples nor thrush are helped by discontinuing nursing; in fact, they may be helped by frequent nursing. Nipple sprays intended to prevent sore nipples (such as Rotersept) have been shown to be ineffective. These Wise Woman preventions and remedies are safe and successful.

Preventing Sore Nipples

• Expose the breasts to air; do not wear a bra all day and all night. Wear your nursing bra with the flaps down whenever possible.

• Expose the breasts to sunlight or brief periods of ultraviolet light (maximum of three minutes, but increase to this level very gradually).

• Rub olive oil, sweet almond oil, lanolin, or Comfrey root ointment into the nipples throughout the latter part of the pregnancy and the beginning weeks of nursing.

• Place the baby correctly, making certain that the entire areola (dark area) is in her/his mouth and that the nipple is centered.

• Experiment with different nursing positions.

• Nurse often so that the baby doesn't get hungry enough to tear at the breast.

• Avoid washing the nipples with soap. Soap removes natural oils and predisposes the nipple to chapping and cracking. Cologne, deodorant, and powder should also be kept away from the nipples.

Remedies for Sore Nipples

• Apply crushed **ice** in a wet cloth or a (wet and) frozen gauze pad to the nipples immediately before nursing. Ice is a good local pain killer; it also helps bring out soft or small nipples or the nipple of a very full breast so the baby can feed more easily.

★ Use **Comfrey root ointment** to soften and strengthen nipples at the same time. Comfrey root ointments are exceptionally soothing to sensitive nipples and rapidly heal any fissures or bruises. Be sure to rinse any ointment off the areola before nursing so the baby can grasp the breast properly.

• Yarrow leaf, poultices or ointment, totally relieves pain and heals cracked nipples rapidly.

• Help heal and strengthen the nipples with **vitamin E**. Apply the oil after nursing. Be sure to use only pure vitamin E, not preparations or synthetics.

• Any of the **poultices** described for painful breasts (pages 86-87) may be used advantageously; Comfrey and Marshmallow are especially effective. Several brief poultices work better than one or two lengthy sessions.

• Apply the clear gel from a fresh **Aloe Vera** leaf to soothe and heal sore and cracked nipples. Be sure to wash it off before nursing as the taste can be quite bitter.

• Try homemade or commercial Calendula ointment to heal and strengthen nipples.

• CAUTION: Ointments containing antibiotics, steroids, and anesthetic (pain-killing) drugs are potentially harmful to you and your infant.

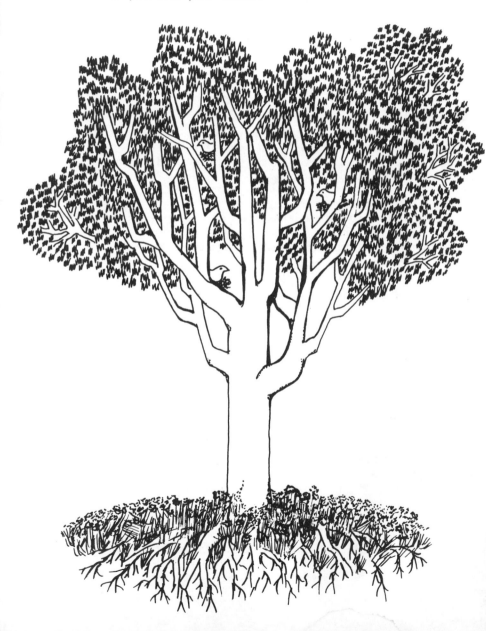

References & Resources

- *The Complete Book of Breastfeeding*
  Sally Olds and Marvin Eiger; 1972, Bantam Books

- *Nursing Your Baby*
  Karen Pryor; 1973, Simon & Schuster

- *The Womanly Art of Breastfeeding*
  LaLeche League; 1963

- *Breastfeeding Basics*
  Cecilia Worth; 1983, McGraw Hill

- LaLeche League
  9616 Minneapolis Avenue, Franklin Park, IL 60131

- *Aftercare;* Sharon Hamilton
- *Babies Grow on Milk and Kisses;* Amy Galblum
  Booklets available from Emma Goldman Clinic for Women
  715 Dodge Street, Iowa City, IA 52240

- *The Way of Herbs*
  Michael Tierra; 1980, Unity Press

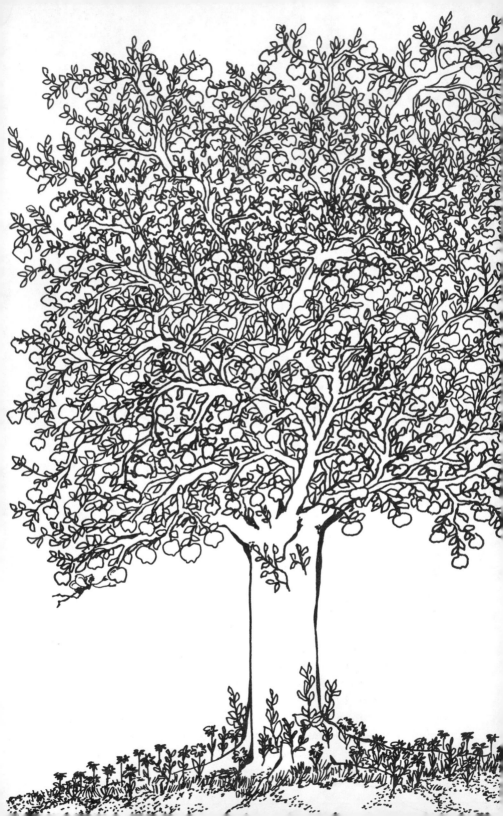

Your Infant

The last two months of the childbearing year focus on your newborn infant, as well as you. Your baby makes tremendous changes as s/he adapts to a new environment and separate existence. Emotional, spiritual, and physical adjustments in your infant's first months include breathing, coping with cold, light, hunger, and loneliness, healing the umbilicus, focusing the eyes, eliminating extra red blood cells, initiating digestive functions, and learning that other beings exist. According to the individual infant, these changes may be trouble-free or troublesome. This chapter shares Wise Woman herbs and remedies which safely and successfully prevent and heal most of the annoying and a few of the frightening problems that your newborn and you will encounter.

No Breath

• **Clear** the infant's **airways** (nose and mouth). Seek immediate assistance if simple wiping and sucking don't remove all mucus or if you see colored mucus.

• Flick your fingertips across the soles of the baby's feet to initiate the gasp reflex.

• Rub Bach **Rescue Remedy** on the newborn's wrists, temples, and lips.

• Use artifical respiration or cardio-pulmonary resuscitation (CPR) as appropriate if there is no response within one minute of the birth. Training in CPR is available through the American Red Cross and the American Heart Association.

• **Don't give up.** Hold your baby close and talk to her, tell her why you want her here or anything else that occurs to you.

Umbilical Care

The cut end of the umbilical cord is a likely entrance for bacteria. Since bacteria prefer airless and damp situations, the usual recommendation is to keep the umbilical stump exposed, dry, and clean until it heals completely and falls off. Allowing your baby to be naked is a highly effective way to insure a dry and airy umbilicus. When you do diaper, be certain that the umbilicus is above the diaper. Wise Woman traditional herbal remedies speed healing and counter infection.

• Use **honey** to coat the umbilical stump. This may seem messy or peculiar to you, but generations of wise bee women swear that it absolutely prevents infection and helps the cord dry fast. Honey is a safe sterile dressing and astringent agent for all wounds and burns, and is a "natural" for umbilical care.

• Apply **Witch Hazel extract,** as it comes from the drugstore, to the umbilicus with a soft cloth. Witch Hazel is a powerful astringent. It closes and dries the stump quickly.

• Expose your naked infant to sunlight for a few minutes every day. Fresh **air and sunlight** are potent healers and perfect infection preventers. If weather prohibits outdoor sunning, lay your infant in a sunny window. See page 103, for further benefits of sunbaths for newborns.

• Brew up **Comfrey leaf compresses** for postpartum care of mother's perineum and infant's umbilicus. Externally, Comfrey soothes torn and cut skin, relieves pain, and promotes very rapid healing. Remember to compress several times a day for no more than five minutes at a time.

• Rosemary leaves   The antiseptic and healing properties of *Rosmarinus officinalis* are strong enough to challenge a mild infection at the umbilical stump. Use Rosemary tincture or powdered Rosemary directly on the umbilicus at every diaper change to quickly dry it and kill the bacteria.

• Echinacea root   Put a drop or two of *Echinacea augustifolia* tincture right on the umbilical stump several times a day to encourage rapid healing, discourage bacteria, and eliminate mild infections. A woman with a colostomy which continued to be mildly infected and raw months after the surgery, says that three drops of Echinacea tincture right on the wound and one night without her bag effected a complete healing.

Also: BLACK SAMPSON, COMB FLOWER, HEDGEHOG, RED SUNFLOWER, KANSAS SNAKE-ROOT, CONEFLOWER

If infection is clearly present, as evidenced by redness, extreme tenderness, or pus, use Echinacea tincture internally to counter it. The usual dose in this case is one drop per pound of body weight given once a day. A crafty mother slips the dropper alongside her nipple and administers the dose while the infant nurses. You can also take Echinacea yourself and give it to your baby through your milk. Drink half a cupful of infusion or a dropperful of tincture in some water fifteen or twenty minutes before nursing, three times daily. Whatever way you administer the Echinacea to counter established infection, continue with it for a minimum of a week or until the infection is completely cleared.

If you think Echinacea is unpronounceable, just call it "E for Emergency."

Circumcision

If you give birth in a hospital in the United States, your baby boy will automatically be circumcised. The procedure involves strapping the baby down and crushing the foreskin off the penis. No painkillers are used. If you don't want your baby circumcised, you may have to arrange it before you enter the hospital. For more information on circumcision, contact INTACT. (See References and Resources.)

Postpartum Eye Care

Last year I saw a film on the life of a blind woman; afterward, she spoke and answered questions. The first question was whether she had been born blind. "Oh, no," she said, "the doctor blinded me with his eye drops."

Silver nitrate drops are routinely (and by law) used in hospitals to prevent possible blindness from gonorrheal infection transferred from the birth canal to the newborn's eyes. Incorrect use can result in blindness. Even correct use is highly irritating to the infant's sensitive eyes. Many midwives do not use silver nitrate, claiming that a serious eye infection is easy to spot and cure and that the irritation from the drops masks the signs of gonorrheal infection on the rare occasions when it does occur.

If you are pregnant and want your baby protected from the physical and emotional trauma of silver nitrate, plan a home birth, and have a culture taken to check for gonorrhea about a month before your due date. (Some midwives advise repeating a negative culture, since they are inaccurate twenty percent of the time.) Use any of the following alternative eye drops, if necessary.

• Neosporin and Illotycin are allopathic antibiotics formulated specifically for babies' eyes and available only by prescription. Neosporin is a penicillin derivatrive and may cause a life-threatening allergic reaction. Illotycin is a form of erythromycin, a different family than penicillin. Both are much less irritating than silver nitrate. Some obstetricians will use these rather than silver nitrate if you state them as your preference.

• **Echinacea,** the herbal antibiotic, is well suited to deal with any bacteria in the eyes of the just born child. Put up an infusion when labor begins and let it steep at room temperature until needed. Strain the infusion carefully through a towel or coffee filter to remove all herbal matter. Use a sterile dropper to put several drops of the infusion into each eye. A dilution of the tincture (5-6 drops in an ounce of water) may also be used but may be slightly irritating.

• An eyewash of **Golden Seal** and **Eyebright** is the herbalists' standard for all eye problems. Brew a half ounce of dried Eyebright and two whole Goldenseal roots in a pint of boiling water for at least eight hours. Strain the brew very thoroughly, through a coffee filter or cotton towel, before storing in your refrigerator or freezer. Avoid Goldenseal powder, as it is very difficult to strain out completely. You can keep this infusion for up to a month if you wish to prepare it well before your due date.

Eye Infections

Common causes of red, stuck together eyelids, and eye irritations in newborns are: blocked tear duct, irritation from silver nitrate or prescription antibiotic drops, yeast infection, inclusion conjunctivitis, gonorrheal infection, and pinkeye.

• Unblock a tear duct and soothe irritations with mild salt water or remedies for pinkeye.

• Use eyewashes of Golden Seal or Red Clover infusion, well strained, for yeast infections.

• Inclusion conjunctivitis is caused by chlamydia bacteria. These bacteria infect the cervixes of about 10% of all

women, usually non-symptomatically. As many as 50% of
the babies born to these women will get inclusion
conjunctivitis. Infection from chlamydia is usually obvious
within a week or two of the birth, but does occasionally
appear as much as six weeks after the birth. Untreated,
inclusion conjunctivitis can lead to permanent scarring of
the conjunctiva. Treatment within fifteen days with
sulfonamides (a prescription drug) is said to clear the
infection and prevent scarring. I have no information on
herbal treatments used successfully with this infection; I
would try Echinacea (of course).

• Gonorrheal infections appear soon after birth, usually
within the first week. An untreated gonorrheal infection in
a newborn's eyes can lead to blindness. This can be
prevented if the infant is treated with antibiotics within
one week.

Pinkeye

Also known as conjunctivitis, pinkeye is a bacterial
infection of the conjunctiva, the lining of the eyelid and
eyeball. It is quite contagious and easily spread through
contact with the exudate (pus) on towels, bedding, and
fingers. Be very careful not to contaminate your own eyes
by thoughtless rubbing, and not to spread the infection
from one of the infant's eyes to the other.

• **Breast milk** is the mothers' and midwives' favorite
curative for pinkeye. For mild infections, use a squirt or
two directly in the eye from the breast. For more
entrenched infections, carefully flush the eye with about a
tablespoon of fresh breast milk at least five times daily.
CAUTION: Do not use this remedy if the mother has
mastitis (breast infection).

★ Chickweed   This common little weed, *Stellaria
media*, grows abundantly around the world, and is my
favorite cure for conjunctivitis. It is so effective when fresh
that the pinkeye is sometimes cleared in one day. Pour
boiling water over a handful of the green stalks, leaves,
and tiny flowers. (If you have only dried Chickweed, soak
it in boiling water for fifteen minutes or until it looks

German:
VOGELMIERE,
HUHNERDARM

French:
STELLAIRE,
MOURON DES
OISEAUX

plump.) Apply the warm plant directly to the eyelid of the afflicted eye(s) and leave it on until it cools. **Throw away the plant material after use.** Depending on the severity of the infection, poultice four to ten times a day. Results are usually immediate and dramatic. Definite clearing should be obvious within 48 hours. Continue poulticing for a day or two after all symptoms are gone to complete the healing and forestall remission.

Also:
STITCHWORT,
SCARWORT,
STAR WEED,
SATIN FLOWER

• Mothers, midwives, and Wise Women herbalists use a great variety of herbs to clear minor eye problems. Those used most often are Golden Seal, Eyebright, and Chamomile. Make a tea of one or more of them, strain carefully, and use the brew to compress or wash your baby's eyes.

• Chinese Wise Women say to lick the newborn's eyes to prevent and cure conjunctivitis. Saliva is most definitely curative and the infection attacks only the eyes, so it is safe to lick it away.

• CAUTION: If you use a remedy for pinkeye and see no improvement within 3 days, seek diagnostic help without delay.

Jaundice

There are three different types of jaundice that your newborn may exhibit, all characterized by a yellow cast in the skin and eyes: physiologic jaundice, breast milk jaundice, and pathological jaundice. Although it may be alarming to see your new baby turn yellow, there is no cause for fear from the first two types of jaundice. Untreated pathological jaundice, however, can lead to *kernicterus* and brain damage. The type of jaundice is determined by the general health of your baby, the level of *bilirubin* in your baby's blood, and how the bilirubin level increases or decreases. Read this entire section through before attempting home treatment of jaundice.

Preventing Jaundice

Here's how jaundice usually happens: Your fetus received oxygen from your placenta. The oxygenated blood from the placenta mixed with the deoxygenated blood of the fetus. To compensate for this mixing, your fetus had a large number of red blood cells. Since your baby was born, s/he has been supplying her/his own oxygen and no longer needs so many red blood cells. The extra red blood cells are broken down by an enzyme produced by your baby's liver. The immature intestines, however, do not fully process out the broken-down red blood cells. Bilirubin, a break-down by-product of this process, thus is reabsorbed and circulates, tinting the skin and eyes yellow.

• Eat a diet rich in minerals, vitamins, and protein while pregnant. Well-nourished mothers bear children with healthy livers, capable of clearing the extra red blood cells more rapidly.

• Include **Dandelion** in your diet throughout your pregnancy and early lactation to help your fetus develop a strong liver. Try Dandelion leaves, cooked or raw, and Dandelion root, tinctured or decocted. Use a tablespoon of decoction or 10 drops of tincture several times a week, or one serving of Dandelion weekly during the last three months of pregnancy. This is especially recommended if you had a previous child with pathological jaundice.

• **Avoid all drugs** during labor. Pitocin, routinely used in hospitals to induce and hasten labor, is known to cause high bilirubin levels. Many allopathic drugs, and stress in general, also slow down the functioning of the newborn's liver and thus increase the duration of jaundice.

• Cut the umbilical cord as soon as practical after the delivery. A long wait forces the newborn to accept more blood and more red blood cells from the placenta.

• **Nurse** your baby **frequently** during the first week. Every four hours is a minimum. Babies who nurse often excrete bilirubin more efficiently and are less likely to be jaundiced. Make certain that you get plenty of liquids to help establish a plentiful supply of breast milk.

• Put your baby's crib in a room with lots of natural light. Babies nearest to the windows in hospitals are the least likely to become jaundiced.

Physiologic Jaundice

Physiologic jaundice is the technical term for the normal jaundice of newborns, which usually appears one to five days after birth. Approximately 70% of all newborns show some physiologic jaundice. Blonds and Native American babies, babies born with the aid of drugs, babies who are not allowed to breast feed at once and on demand, and premature babies are at greatest risk of developing severe physiologic jaundice. The symptoms are yellow skin, yellow eyes, a bilirubin level of 12 or more which decreases soon after the third day, and an active baby. If your baby is nursing well, you may safely treat physiologic jaundice at home. The rule here is: "A healthy acting yellow baby is a healthy baby." Normal jaundice generally disappears within a week.

• **Nurse, nurse, nurse.** Your breast milk, especially your first milk, colostrum, helps your baby colonize the intestinal bacteria s/he needs to help bind and excrete the broken down red blood cells. Nursing also provides her/him with extra protein, which protects the brain from damage while the bilirubin level is high. Nurse immediately. Nurse often.

• Undress your baby, cover her/his eyes, and put her/him in the sun every day. **Sunlight** breaks down bilirubin. Five minutes of early morning or late afternoon sunlight, even filtered through clouds or glass, is the recommended minimum. Continue the sunbaths for at least a week, or until your baby's skin returns to its normal tone.

• Sip **Catnip tea** and offer some to your baby. Appalachian midwives favor the wild Catmint for controlling jaundice and report complete success when the mother consumes at least two cups a day, preferably just prior to nursing.

• Supplement your scant breast milk during the first few days with **Comfrey leaf tea** for your baby. Comfrey has become a controversial herb recently and many mothers are afraid to give it to their infants. The problematic factor is found only in fresh young Comfrey; a tea of dried leaves is safe and beneficial. In fact, Comfrey leaf contains several amino acids necessary for proper brain growth of fetuses and babies. It also helps colonize the intestines of the newborn with beneficial bacteria.

German:
ODERMENNING

French:
AIGREMOINE

Also:
COCKLEBURR,
STICKLEWORT,
BURR MARIGOLD

• Help resolve jaundice with **Agrimony infusions.** This fairly easily found weed grows all over the world and is a Wise Woman choice for correcting liver, gall bladder, spleen, and kidney problems. Pick the whole plant while it is flowering and dry it well. Half a cup of the pleasant, but astringent, brew will pass its effect through the breast milk to the jaundiced baby if taken several times daily just prior to nursing.

• Enlist the aid of Dandelion if your newborn's jaundice is severe. Sip **Dandelion root infusion** or decoction throughout the day. The brew is bitter but tolerable if salt (not sweet) is added to it. Drops of the infusion or decoction can also be given directly to your infant. Either way, directly or through your breast milk, Dandelion stimulates and supports powerful liver functioning in the newborn. There is no limit to the amount of Dandelion you can use (except the taste); the daily minimum is one cup of the infusion for you, or one teaspoon of the decoction for your baby.

Breast Milk Jaundice

This jaundice usually appears sometime after the first two weeks of your baby's life. It is quite rare, occurring in only 0.5% of all newborns. Its symptoms are yellow skin, yellow eyes, a bilirubin level of up to 20, and an active, nursing baby. As its name implies, this jaundice is caused by breast milk. It is thought that steroids in breast milk occasionally act as an antagonist to the enzymes that break down the extra red blood cells in the infant. Breast milk jaundice often persists for as long as two months.

• **Relax.** There is no real need to treat breast milk jaundice if your baby is healthy, active, and nursing strongly.

• **Cheladonium 3x** is the homeopathic remedy for all types of jaundice. The energy from the brilliant yellow flowers and orange sap of this weed can help stimulate strong liver functioning. CAUTION: Do not use the herb Cheladonium (Celandine) itself, only the homeopathic essence or the flower essence.

• Stop feeding breast milk for a very short while, no more than 48 hours, if your infant gets yellower and yellower and you suspect breast milk jaundice. If there is true breast milk jaundice, the bilirubin level will drop 5-10 points. Resume nursing immediately. There is no reason to stop nursing altogether; in fact, it may complicate the jaundice if you remove the nurturing closeness of breast feeding.

• Increase enzymatic activity in your baby's liver and intestines with small amounts of fresh Wheat grass juice. (See page 39.) Your baby may take up to 20 drops daily. If you prefer to pass the benefit along in your milk, work your way up to drinking two ounces daily. Large amounts of this chlorophyll concentrate can cause minor side effects such as nausea.

Pathological Jaundice

Pathological jaundice occurs due to pathological processes in your newborn, such as an Rh or ABO blood group incompatibility, or a damaged or malformed liver, or as a side effect of several maternal conditions, including drug use. This jaundice appears within the first week of life, often by the first day. Symptoms include yellow skin and eyes, a bilirubin level of 12 or more which *continues to rise* after the third day, and a dehydrated, lethargic baby. CAUTION: It is not advisable to treat pathological jaundice at home without the aid of an experienced professional healer. Untreated pathological jaundice can lead to brain damage.

Colic

Listening to the howling screams of my colicky baby was one of my worst ordeals as a new mother. Your baby's digestive system is not fully developed at birth. Colic (severe abdominal pain) is caused by spasmodic contractions of immature intestines or gas trapped in the intestines. Be aware that your child's digestion is strongly affected by you. Your emotions, the foods you eat (if you are nursing), your sense of security and well-being, and other individual factors contribute to the presence or absence of colic. Use these remedies in any order; they are all safe, gentle, and effective.

Preventing Colic, General

• Feed your baby often. **Small, frequent feedings** are less likely to produce colic than a few large ones.

• Soothe your infant with **skin-to-skin contact** during feedings. This is reassuring to your child and promotes good digestion.

• Try the **"colic hold"** recommended by the LaLeche League. Hold your baby astraddle your arm with the head resting in the crook of your elbow and the top of the legs in your hand. Be sure the head stays higher than the feet while the baby nurses.

Preventing Colic, Breast-fed Babies

• Do not eat cabbage family plants (broccoli, brussels sprouts, turnips, radishes, kale, collards, cauliflower, and all types of cabbage), onions or garlic during the first six months of your lactation. All these foods are rich in sulphur which promotes intestinal gas in you and your baby.

• Avoid more than one small glass of prune juice daily. Any laxatives may distress your infant's intestines.

• Avoid chocolate, peanuts, peanut butter, sugar, and white flour. All of these foods disrupt and slow intestinal activity in you and your baby.

• Eliminate possible allergens from your diet. Allergies to soy, wheat, corn, dairy, and pectin (in most fruit) can cause colic.

• Nurse in a serene, secure environment. If you can't provide it physically, create it mentally.

Preventing Colic, Bottle-fed Babies

• Use **goat milk,** if available, for your bottle-fed baby. Remember how well "Heidi" did on goat milk and fresh air. Cow milk contains seven times as much casein (a protein) as human milk, and very large fat globules, both of which can be difficult to digest and gas forming. Also, the low lactose content of cow milk makes it difficult for the proper digestive bacteria (lactobacillus) to thrive in the baby's intestines, making colic even more likely. Goat milk has the same amount of casein as human milk, very small fat globules, and a high lactose content.

• Add **acidophilus** to cow milk if you can't get fresh goat milk. Use a tablespoon of acidophilus liquid or a capsule of the powder (open it and pour the powder into the formula) in every eight ounce bottle to make the cow milk more digestible. If acidophilus is unavailable, substitute a tablespoon of fresh yogurt.

Remedies For Colic

• Use **aromatic seeds,** such as Fennel, Dill, Caraway, Anise, Cumin, or Coriander to prevent and relieve colic. Drink a cup of seed tea as you settle down to nurse; the antispasmodic and *carminative* effects pass readily into your breast milk. Or give your baby a bottle of seed tea to suck on. Prepare seed tea by pouring one cup of boiling water over a scant teaspoon of any one of the seeds. Steep for no more than fifteen minutes. Strain very thoroughly before filling baby's bottle. Try seed teas warm or chilled. (See Appendix II - Nursing Formula.)

Spanish:
YERBA GATERA,
NEBADA

German:
KATZENMINZE

French:
NÉPÉTA DES CHATS

Chinese:
CHI·HSUEH·TS'AO

Also:
CATMINT, CAT'S
WORT, CATNEP

• Appalachian midwives swear by **Catnip** tea for colicky babies. It relieves spasms in the intestines and encourages sleep. One of my friends uses it to put her baby to sleep when he is especially cranky and reports that it works very well indeed.

• Put cold wet wool socks on your baby's feet when s/he has colic. Pull dry cotton socks on over the wool ones. Your infant should relax and fall asleep quickly. I don't understand how this works; it sounds strange, but sleepless mothers acclaim it.

Also:
RED ELM,
MOOSE ELM,
INDIAN ELM

★ Slippery Elm bark   You might think of tree bark as tough and terrible tasting, but the inner bark of *Ulmus fulva* is one of the most soothing of all herbs to the digestive system, and it tastes rather like maple syrup. Every time I've encountered an infant with severe colic or allergic reactions to food, Slippery Elm has restored digestive stability and strength. Although no nutritional breakdown of this herb is available, Native Americans consider it alone adequate as an emergency foodstuff, and I have seen babies thrive on it as their primary nourishment for weeks at a time when they could tolerate no other food.

The basic preparation is as a "gruel," rather than a tea, for Slippery Elm is so slippery that the tea resembles snot! Make the gruel by mixing a liquid sweetener (such as barley malt, sorghum, or maple syrup) with Slippery Elm powder, until it is all wet. Then add hot milk or water slowly until a slippery porridge results. (Do not feed honey to children younger than one year old. Botulinus spores, non-harmful to adults, may be present in the honey and cause botulism, a sometimes fatal illness, in an infant.) You can also prepare Slippery Elm by adding it when you make hot cereals. Replace a spoonful or two of the dry cereal with Slippery Elm powder, then cook your cereal as usual.

There is no known limit to the amount of Slippery Elm that can safely be consumed. For colic, add one or more servings of Slippery Elm to the diet to help quiet the intestines. In severe cases, give your infant only Slippery Elm for several days, then gradually resume normal feedings.

Thrush

Candida albicans is a yeast which is a normal *symbiotic* part of our bodies. It can reproduce wildly during times of stress, colonizing the vagina, intestines, throat, mouth, nipples and arm folds. In the vagina, it is known as a yeast infection, or the whites, or leukorrhea. If it overruns the intestines, it causes food allergies and low resistance to disease. When it establishes itself in the throat and mouth or arm folds of an infant, or on the nipples of a nursing mother, it is called thrush.

Thrush is a prime suspect if your baby seems hungry but fusses instead of nursing. Look inside the infant's mouth. Are the insides of the cheeks and the throat redder than normal? Check carefully for white patches on the inner cheeks and other tender tissue; these are yeast colonies. On the nipples or in the arm folds the thrush will cause flaky, red, sore, crepy looking skin.

These remedies offer several excellent ways of dealing with thrush. When they are successful, the thrush will diminish or disappear within three days, but you will have to continue using them for weeks to completely clear out the thrush and forestall a reoccurrence. All are equally strong.

• In addition to any remedy, take special care with **hygiene** to keep the thrush from spreading. Wash your hands every time you use the bathroom, touch the baby's mouth, or touch your nipples.

• Coat the inside of your baby's mouth with **yogurt** after each feeding. Bread bakers know that yeast grows very poorly in the presence of yogurt, and thousands of women have testified to the effectiveness of yogurt for curing vaginal yeast infections. Homemade yogurt is the optimum, acidophilus yogurt is a good second best, but practically any yogurt will do. Dip your finger in the yogurt and offer it to be sucked; wash your finger afterward. Or smear the yeast patches with yogurt on a cotton swab, and discard the swab. Or freeze small cubes of yogurt and let your baby mouth them; clean up carefully. Also smear your nipples with yogurt; wash before nursing. Take special care not to contaminate your yogurt with thrush.

• Dissolve a level teaspoon of baking soda in eight ounces of water. Using a fresh cotton swab thoroughly wipe the insides of the baby's cheeks, the gums, and the tongue with this solution after every nursing. Prepare the solution fresh every day and stir well before using. Discourage thrush on your nipples by bathing them after nursing with a **vinegar** solution made from one tablespoon vinegar in a cup of water. This need not be made fresh every day.

• Soak **Plantain seeds** in just enough water to cover them until they swell (overnight), then put the gel-like brew onto the white patches of thrush. Said to be a specific for thrush, Plantain seeds (*Plantago major*) are easily gathered in the fall. If you haven't harvested any, Psyllium seed (*Plantago ovata* and *P. psyllium*) may be available commercially. All types of Plantain seeds are very sticky and *mucilaginous*.

• Prepare a tea using a half teaspoon **Golden Seal powder** to a cup of boiling water. A dose of the well-stirred, room temperature tea is one half teaspoonful per ten pounds of body weight, two to three times a day. Working topically in the mouth, and throughout the whole system, Golden Seal destroys yeast colonies. I'd try this only as a last resort, because infants routinely reject the robustly bitter and long lasting taste of *Hydrastis canadensis*. CAUTION: Golden Seal can destroy beneficial intestinal bacteria and cause diarrhea and increase colic distress if used excessively.

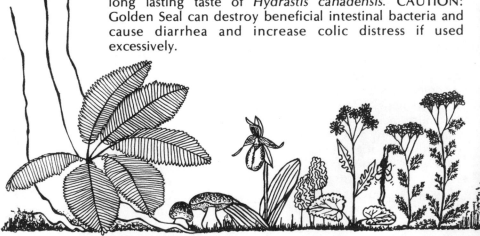

Diaper Rash

I've yet to meet a mother or child who didn't have to deal with diaper rash at some time. The causes of diaper rash are varied; they include yeast infection, irritation from paper diapers, generally sensitive skin, reaction to the soap used to wash the diapers, digestive disturbance from some food that the nursing mother has eaten, and reaction to antibiotic drugs. These remedies range from mild to strong.

Preventing Diaper Rash

• The ultimate prevention (and cure) for diaper rash is to **eliminate diapers!**

Mothers in Uganda carry their undiapered babies slung to their bare breasts. They say it is easy to know when the child is about to "soil" and claim never to be wet or shat on. Many mothers have noticed that their infants have predictable bowel movements associated with nursing.

Absorbent materials may be laid under the sleeping infant. Sphagnum moss is notably absorbent. Cattail down was a favorite of many American Indian women. The easiest, though costly, modern diaper replacement is a cradle liner of sheepskin, which will absorb much moisture and can be laundered easily. (One mother pointed out that the cost of the sheepskin was not more than the cumulative cost of washing cloth diapers or buying disposable ones, and that it made a wonderful rug after its diaper-duty days were done.)

• **Change diapers promptly** after a bowel movement and rinse the baby's bottom with clean water, remembering to dry it well.

• Pay special attention on **wash day** to help prevent diaper rash. Use soap flakes or Basic-H rather than detergent, ammonia, and bleach. Add apple cider vinegar to the final rinse and dry diapers in the sunlight whenever possible.

• Use **Arrowroot powder** or **clay powder** rather than talc or commercial baby powders. Talc is considered a cancer-causing agent; scented commercial powders can cause rashes.

• Use olive oil, wheat germ oil, **Plantain oil,** or other simple oils instead of lotions or vaseline. Lotions are usually scented and liable to cause reactions on sensitive skins; vaseline (and mineral oil) is a petroleum by-product which interferes with the natural absorption of oil-soluble vitamins A, D, and E.

• Avoid plastic pants over diapers. They save the bedclothes but promote diaper rash. **Wool soakers** are a good alternative. If you do elect to use plastic pants, limit the time you have them on your baby as much as possible.

Remedies for Diaper Rash

• Harness the curative properties of **sunlight!** Even stubborn cases of diaper rash clear when your baby's bottom and genitals are exposed to sunlight every day. Outdoors and naked for hours is most effective but even five minutes of sunlight through a window will work.

Spanish: LANTÉN

Gr: WEGERICH

French: PLANTAIN

Chinese: CHÉ CH'IEN

Russian: PODOROSHNIK *'along the road'*

Also: WHITE MAN'S FOOT, WAYBROD, RIPPLE GRASS, PSYLLIUM, WAGBREAD, RIB· WORT, RIBGRASS

★ Plantain   This weed which lines walkways and driveways and pokes through the cracks of city sidewalks is the bane of diaper rash. Use fresh leaves, dried leaves, oil, or ointment of *Plantago* to heal and relieve the pain and itching of diaper rash. Both broad (*P. major*) and narrow (*P. lanceolata*) leafed varieties are used. Crush clean fresh Plantain leaves and put them next to your baby's skin with each diaper change. Soak dried leaves in hot water until they are soft and use them as an overnight poultice. Directions for making Plantain oil and ointment are in Appendix II.

• Treat diaper rash with a paste of Slippery Elm powder and honey.

Also: KNITBONE, NIP BONE, BONESET, BRUISEWORT, HEALING PLANT, KNITBACK, SLIPPERY ROOT, CONSOLIDA

★ Comfrey root ointment   Allantoin, concentrated in *Symphytum* roots, causes rapid regeneration of skin cells and is a noted healer of all wounds, irritations, and rashes. In an oil base, Comfrey root soothes, heals, and strengthens the skin so it is less likely to be abraded or irritated. Prepare your own Comfrey root ointment, buy one already made, or poultice with freshly grated Comfrey root.

Ointments containing Golden Seal or Comfrey leaves (instead of root) are less useful. Golden Seal may further irritate sensitive genitals. Comfrey leaves are not as rich in allantoin as the roots and are less effective against diaper rash.

Yeast Infection Diaper Rash

The most persistent diaper rashes are often traced to a yeast (or fungus) infection in the genital skin folds.

• Avoid using cornstarch as a diapering powder; although it is a recommended substitute for commercial powders, it can encourage yeast growth on some babies' bottoms.

• Avoid giving your baby antibiotics or any food that loosens her/his bowels. Any disruption in the intestines can support yeast growth on the genitals.

• All of the suggestions for thrush (pages 109-110) are applicable, with appropriate modifications. Treat your baby to careful hygiene, yogurt sitz baths, vinegar after-bath anointments, Golden Seal baby powder, and Plantain seed or leaf poultices.

• Cut off the oxygen supply to the yeast by completely coating your baby's diaper rash with egg white, a loose slip of clay, or Slippery Elm gruel. Allow the application to air dry before diapering, or dispense with diapers for a while. Reapply as needed. Look for results within a day or two.

• Use of zinc ointment and epsom salt baths speeds healing of yeast diaper rashes.

• Avoid sources of yeast in your diet if you are breast feeding and yeast diaper rash is a persistent problem. Yeasts are used to ferment wine, beer, and all other spirits, including vinegar. Yeasts raise dough to make bread products. The skins of all fruits and vegetables are usually rich in wild yeasts. Since a low yeast diet is difficult to maintain and balance, discontinue unless your baby shows positive response within two weeks.

Cradle Cap

Apparently caused by overactive sweat or oil glands on the infant's scalp, cradle cap is a yellowish, oily, sometimes scaly crust on the scalp. It is neither serious nor contagious, and need not be treated.

• Apply any type of food **oil** to your baby's scalp and leave it on overnight. This will loosen the cradle cap and you can gently remove the crust the next day. If the cradle cap is extensive, oil and remove a little at a time. Follow each oil treatment with a thorough washing.

• Rub Oak bark infusion, Witch Hazel bark infusion, or black tea into your infant's scalp several times a day, massaging well each time. The **astringent tannins** help slow down the overproduction of oil.

• **Amino-pon soap** is a modern addition to the list of remedies for cradle cap. Use it to wash your baby's scalp thoroughly. It will loosen the cradle cap and allow you to remove the crust.

Also:
CUCKOO BUTTONS,
LOVE LEAVES,
HARE·LOCK, CLOT·
BUR, PERSONATA,
HAPPY MAJOR,
BARDONA,
FOX'S CLOTE

• Use tincture of **Burdock root** to balance the oil production from the scalp. *Arctium* species beneficially influence the oil (sebaceous) and sweat (sudoriferous) glands, especially those in the scalp. The action is tonic; give it to your baby daily for at least three weeks for maximum effect. Infants up to 20 pounds can take 5 drops a day in a bottle of juice or water; infants over 20 pounds can take 10 or more drops daily.

• Relieve cradle cap problems quickly with 2-5 drops of **Wild Pansy** leaf and flower **tincture** given daily for up to a week. This beautiful little flower is widely cultivated and known as Heart's Ease or Johnny Jump-up.

Infections and Fevers

Systemic infection, such as pneumonia, is a frightening and threatening health crisis. The body's natural defense against infection is fever, but very young children tend to run high fevers. A high fever increases the possibility of convulsions. Most parents go right to a doctor. I've worked with some who chose differently. And I trust more than ever that herbal medicines are potent healers.

Preventing Infections

• Use **Echinacea tincture** to prevent infections from exposure to bacteria and viruses in the hospital, contagious fevers, flus, and colds in the family, deep or dirty wounds, and insect bites. A dose of 5-15 drops taken two or three times daily by the nursing mother will pass through the breast milk to protect the infant. If dosing the baby directly, use 1-2 drops twice a day to help prevent infection. See Appendix II for directions for making Echinacea tincture.

Treating Infections with Echinacea

I have seen babies as young as three days old successfully clear serious systemic infections with the assistance of love and breast milk from a mother drinking Echinacea infusions. Older infants as well respond exceptionally favorably to Echinacea. I have seen children a year or more old, who have been on antibiotics since birth, finally regain health after two courses of Echinacea.

The action of Echinacea is quite different than the action of allopathic antibiotics and other antibiotic herbs such as Golden Seal, which directly attack the virus or bacteria and actually weaken the body as a whole. Echinacea vitalizes and strengthens the body's immune system: thymus, adrenals, and lymph glands. It is precisely this ability to generally stimulate and support the immune system that makes Echinacea so valuable as a preventative and a curative for all types of infections.

Echinacea is also a fine fever herb. It does not interfere with the needed elevation of temperature (bacteria and viruses cannot thrive above 100°F), but keeps the fever low enough to prevent convulsions.

I have not observed any side effects or allergic reactions after a decade of using and recommending Echinacea. (Other herbalists report occasional mild stomach upsets.) Echinacea, because it does not directly

kill bacteria, rarely disrupts the intestinal flora and does not encourage diaper rash and yeast infections (as most other antibiotics do). As a further benefit, it is unlikely that viruses will mutate to nullify the effect of Echinacea as they are now doing in response to "wonder drugs." Echinacea has been used for thousands of years by Wise Women to treat cancer, septic conditions, poisonous bites, and severe infections; it still works, and having seen the power of this root, I use it with confidence in the worst situations.

• Infuse *Echinacea augustifolia* root in water to derive the utmost medicinal effect. Two cups of the infusion (one ounce of root steeped for eight hours in a pint of water) daily is the dose for a person weighing 125-150 pounds. When dealing with acute infection, the full dose must be taken for a minimum of seven days, though results will be evident within 48 hours. For a child, give at least two tablespoons of the infusion daily for every ten pounds of body weight.

    You can take (or give) more Echinacea if desired, as there seems to be no reasonable amount that would be an overdose. I usually limit a course of Echinacea to two weeks and repeat it if necessary after a break of two weeks. Entrenched infections and infections which have been treated with repeated doses of allopathic antibiotics often require two or more courses of Echinacea infusions.

    It is not so much the taste as the feeling of Echinacea in the mouth that makes infants reject it. Tincture squirted directly into the mouth produces distressing tingling and numbing sensations. Instead, add the tincture to a small amount of milk, water, or juice and then administer the diffused dose from an eyedropper, spoon, or bottle.

Fever Remedies

There are many, many fever herbs. These are the ones I consider most effective and safe for infants. They lower the temperature without producing a drenching sweat. All are equally effective, but Elder is my favorite.

• Squeeze a whole **lemon** into a cup of very hot water. Add maple syrup if desired. Strain carefully to remove all the lemon pulp and offer it to your infant in a bottle. This "herb" is widely available, rich in infection-fighting vitamin C, and a prompt cooler and rehydrator when fever rises.

• Soak a linen or cotton kitchen towel in apple cider vinegar and place it around your baby's feet. This keeps fevers below the convulsing range.

• Offer a bottle of **Spearmint** or Peppermint **infusion** to your feverish babe. Both Mints are a little too strong for really tiny infants, but they are often available in grocery stores and they cool fevers quickly. You can pass the benefit on through your breast milk, too.

• Say "E for Emergency" and put 10 drops of **Echinacea tincture** in a four ounce bottle of water. Allow your baby to suck this as desired to keep the fever within bounds. A feverish and delirious two-year-old went to sleep after drinking half a glass of tincture water; she awoke cool, easy, and asking for "more funny water."

★ Elder   The fragile, cream-colored flowers of *Sambucus* species, when tinctured, provide a superb remedy for treating infants' fevers. Elder blossom tincture seems to encourage balance in the mechanism which regulates temperature. It reduces frighteningly high fevers without fail. Put one drop per pound of body weight directly under your baby's tongue, or slide the dropper alongside your nipple and administer the drops while the baby is nursing. (Measure the drops into a spoon, then take the correct dose into the empty dropper.) The dose may be repeated as often as needed; it is completely harmless. The fever usually begins to decrease within a few hours of the first dose.

Spanish: SAUCO

German: SCHWARZER HOLUNDER

French: SUREAU NOIR

        Stories abound about the dangerous Elder. And there is a story told all over the world, in different cultures and various versions, of the woman who lives in the Elder. Sometimes she is called the Elder Lady, sometimes Elder Woman, but my favorite name for her is Elda Mor.
        The stories say that Elda Mor is a Wise Woman who has taken the shape of a tree in order to heal her children. She is powerful and she demands respect. If you wish to have her help, you must honor her. If you abuse her, or

fail to ask her permission to take part of her, Elda Mor will poison you.

Elder grows somewhere near you; look and ask for her. When you find an Elder bush, develop a relationship with Elda Mor. Visit with her from time to time. Then, when the Elder blooms, go out in the moonlight and tell her of your desire to heal with her magic and her knowledge. She will respond, granting permission for you to take her sweet flowers. Thank her and put up your tincture immediately, capturing moon beams, Elder dreams, and the ancient wisdom of women in your bottle.

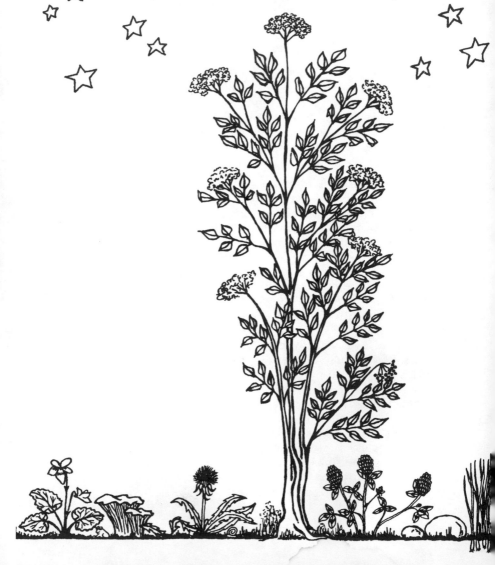

References & Resources

- *Nature's Children*
  Juliette de Bairacli Levy; 1970, Schocken Books

- *Healing the Family*
  Joy Gardner; 1982, Bantam Books

- *Up-to-date Medical Information for the Home*
  Philip Skraina, MD; 1937, Tudor Publishing

- *Feed Your Kids Right*
  Lendon Smith, MD; 1979, Dell Trade Paperbacks

- *Childhood Diseases*
  John Christopher; 1978, Christopher Publications

- *Touching: The Human Significance of Skin*
  Ashley Montagu; 1971, Columbia University Press

- *Mothering* Magazine
  PO Box 2208, Albuquerque, NM 87103

- *Dissatisfied Parents Together News*
  Information packet on vaccines: $3
  128 Branch Rd., Vienna, VA 22180

- *Circumcision: The Painful Dilemma*
  Rosemary Romberg; 1985
  INTACT, 4521 Fremont St., Bellingham, WA 98226

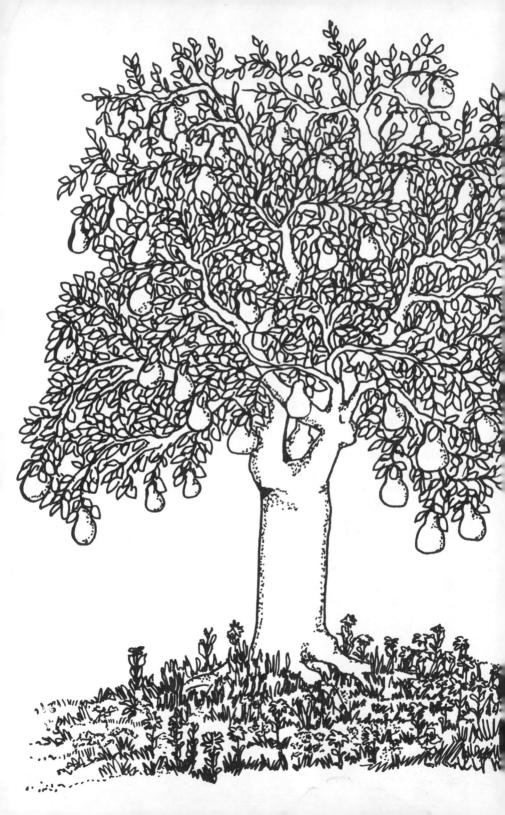

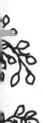

Herbal Pharmacy

In your herbal pharmacy you transform fresh and dried plants into herbal medicines. Learning to identify and use the common plants around you is easy and exciting, beneficial and safe. Making your own medicines saves you money if you follow the Wise Woman tradition of using local herbs, free for the taking. Even one day's work in field, forest, and kitchen can provide you with many years' worth of medicines. When you make your own, you know for sure what's in it, where it came from, when and how it was harvested, and how fresh and potent it is.

Dried herbs are best for the infusions recommended in this book. Stock your herbal pharmacy with your own foraged or cultivated dried herbs; expand your resources and experiment with new herbs by buying dried herbs from reputable sources.

Fresh herbs are best for the tinctures and oils recommended in this book. If you can't make your own, buy from sources who wildcraft or grow their own herbs to use fresh in preparations. Whether you buy or make your medicines, remember, **herbal remedies may not work or may work incorrectly if they aren't prepared correctly.** Read this chapter carefully; it contains easy to follow instructions for every remedy and preparation mentioned in this book.

Meeting the Plants

Start by noticing the plants that live with you, along your driveway or sidewalk. Don't assume that medicinal plants are hard to find. Fennel, Pepper Grass, Dandelion, Plantain, and Mugwort (to name only a few) are as common in cities and suburbs as in the country.

Learn more about the weeds around you directly from the plants, from a personal guide, and from field guides and herbals.

When we open all our senses, including the psychic ones, to the green world, we learn to hear and understand plant language. Through shape, color, location, scent, texture, taste, and energy, plants tell us how they will affect our bodies, which plant parts we can use, and how we can prepare them. Some Wise Women converse with the plant fairies and the *devas*. Some hear the song that each plant sings. Some feel the dances of the leaves, breezes, and insects. All are means of learning the ways of herbs. Though the scientific tradition scoffs at such knowledge, the Wise Woman tradition honors the plant as the ultimate authority on its uses.

A personal guide into the plant world will show you plant features which ensure positive identification, such as the hairs on Wild Carrot which safely distinguish it from Poison Hemlock. A personal guide will introduce you to the foods, medicines, dyes, fibers, decorations, and delights hidden in common plants, and instruct you in wise harvesting and preparation. Check local garden clubs, botanical gardens, and nature centers for contacts with personal guides.

Field guides are indispensable references once your taste for herbal identification is whetted. I find the line drawings in the Peterson guides more helpful than color photographs when I have to distinguish between similar looking plants.

Herbals concentrate on the specifics of using plants as medicines and are rarely illustrated well enough to serve as a guide to identification. Field guides hardly ever include information on medicinal value. The link between your field guide and your herbal is the botanical binomial, or Latin name, of each plant. The binomial is (usually) consistent in all references, unlike common names which overlap and vary from region to region. Once you have identified a new plant, you can look it up by finding the binomial in herbals and other references. This can increase your confidence and ability to find and use safe herbal medicines.

My years of leading Weed Walks and helping people identify wild plants have shown me that learning to recognize herbs in the field is far easier, and much less fraught with danger, than most people realize. As Euell Gibbons is quoted as saying: "You don't learn all the plants at once; you learn them one at a time."

Even if you never pick your own herbs, knowing how the live plants look will be a great asset when you go out to buy them.

Picking Herbs

When you have positively identified the plant you wish to use, center yourself by sitting next to the herb in silence. Take several deep breaths. Feel the earth under you, connecting you to all the plants. Listen to the sounds and songs all around you. Can you hear the song of your herb?

If you are picking only one plant, ask that plant to give you its power. Tell it how you intend to use it. If you are harvesting many plants, look for a grandmother plant. Ask her permission to use her grandchildren. Visualize clearly how you intend to use the plants.

Make an offering of corn or tobacco, a coin or love to the plants. Sing with them. Talk with them if you feel moved to do so. Thank the earth and begin your gathering.

Take care to preserve and contribute to the well-being of the plant community. Take no more than half of the annuals or biennials, no more than a third of the perennials. Walk gently and with balance.

Harvest plants when the energy you want is most concentrated. Roots store energy in the form of sugar, starch, and medicinal alkaloids throughout the cold or dormant season; pick them when above ground growth of the plant has died back. Leaves process energy to nourish roots and flowers; pick them at their most lush, before flowers have formed, after all dew has dried, and before the day's heat wilts them. Flowers are fragile, pollen-filled, joyous; harvest them in full bloom, before seeds form, and before bees visit them. Seeds are durable, but likely to shatter and disperse if left on the plant too long; harvest seeds when still green and before insects invade. Barks (inner barks and root barks) may be harvested at any time but are thought to be most potent in spring and fall. Look carefully at the plant you wish to pick and you will see where the energy is highest; let this guide your harvesting.

Deal with your harvest immediately. Allowing the cut plants to lie about dissipates their vital energies, encourages mold and fermentation, and results in poor quality preparations. If you intend to eat your harvest, refrigerate the plants, or wash and cook them and sit down and eat. If you intend to make a tincture or oil, cover the herbs with alcohol or oil as soon as possible; don't refrigerate

them. If you intend to dry the herbs, it is vital to lay them out or tie
them up as soon after harvest as possible.

Drying Herbs

To dry herbs and maintain their color, fragrance, taste, energy, and
medicinal potency, you need only:
  • Pick when there is no moisture on the plant and do not wash
the plant (roots are the exception).
  • Dry the herbs immediately after picking, in small bunches or
spread out so parts don't touch.
  • Dry them in a dark and well-ventilated area.
  • Take down the herbs and store in paper bags as soon as they
are crisply dried. If insect invasions force you to store dried herbs in
glass or plastic, air-dry them, then dry in paper bags for another two
weeks before sealing in tight containers.
  • Keep the herbs as whole, cool, and dark as possible during
storage. Under optimum storage conditions, well-dried volatile,
delicate herbs last about six months; roots and barks maintain
potency for six or more years.

Problems with Foraging

Are you concerned about contamination of wild plants with lead,
chemicals, and dog doo?
  Avoid harvesting herbs from roadsides where lead concentration
is high; plants growing by busy roads will accumulate more lead.
The nearer the plant is to the road, the higher the level of lead
concentration. If you can't find a particular herb anywhere except
by a road, pick at least eight feet from the road edge; lead levels
drop sharply in the first few feet. In cities, pick from parks and
other out-of-the-way places. Be wary of vacant lots which may be
contaminated with lead paint.
  Avoid picking under powerlines and along roads where the
weeds are controlled by spraying instead of cutting. Suburban
lawns that have been doused with weed killers rarely grow
medicinal weeds, but if you suspect chemical warfare (distorted,
mutated, sparse weeds are good clues), avoid that area.
  Avoid gathering herbs where canines gather. Dogs can pass
parasites to humans.
  Allow yourself to be guided by your intuition, as well as your
senses and your intelligence, and you will know which areas to
avoid when picking wild plants. Given the amount of chemical

contamination on commercial herbs (and fruits and vegetables, for that matter), I honestly feel safer taking risks in the wild.

Open your eyes and observe the green abundance. Open your heart and feel the green joy. Come with respect for green power. The devas of the plant kingdom welcome you.

Buying Herbs

Knowing how to buy herbs is a necessary skill, just like learning to identify them. It is my personal goal to find or grow all the herbs I use. But even with access to a garden and hundreds of acres of Catskill country, I haven't yet achieved my goal. I, too, buy herbs collected, grown, and prepared by others.

In the last few years I have become aware of many practices in the commercial herb trade which appall me. Grossly substandard wages are paid to harvesters in Third World countries. Pesticide and herbicide chemicals banned in the United States are used on herbs grown overseas (and 80% of commercial herbs are imported). Dried herbs may be legally irradiated with the equivalent of hundreds of chest X-rays, yet there is no labeling as to which herbs have been so treated. All commercial herbal warehouses, even those storing organic herbs, must legally be fumigated several times a year with chemical sprays.

I protect myself by purchasing herbs from individuals I know and trust. Their names and addresses are included in the References and Resources following this chapter.

Whatever the source, dried herbs should be brightly colored, fresh smelling, and as whole as possible. Powdered herbs and herbs in capsules lose medicinal value rapidly, with some exceptions, like Ginger, Slippery Elm, and Golden Seal.

When you look at a dried herb, envision it as it was when alive. The only thing that should be missing is the water content. Red Clover blossoms are a vibrant purplish-pink, not brown. Raspberry leaves are white on one side and green on the other, not a uniform brown. Witch Hazel bark shows the lighter color of the *cambium* along with the darker grey of the bark; it doesn't look like leftovers from the wood pile.

Smell dried herbs carefully and reject those which lack scent and those which smell of chemicals or molds. Peppermint and Licorice, for instance, should fill your head with their scent. Comfrey root should smell clean and fresh, not musty and moldy.

The energy, or life force, of an herb can be sensed even when the plant has been dried. Absence of energy means that the herb is old, or has been handled incorrectly. If you can, hold the dried herb in your hands: feel for tingle, look for sparkle. A pendulum will react to the life force present in dried herbs; dowsing can confirm your sensory impressions.

If you are buying by mail, return herbs that do not look, smell, and feel alive. If you buy from a store, bring poor quality to the attention of the owner and demand unpowdered and unencapsulated herbs. Say what you want and what pleases you. Consumer desires do have power in the herb market. Interest in organically grown herbs has resulted in increased availability of organic medicinals.

Making Herbal Medicines

The art of making herbal preparations is fascinating and complex. Each herb has one or more optimum methods of preparation, each method extracting different properties from the herb. Each type of preparation affects the body in different ways. The quality of herbal preparation is dependent on the quality of the herb used. The quality of the herb is affected by the weather during the growing season, the thoughts of the gatherer or grower, when the herb is harvested, and the conditions surrounding handling and storage. The moon sheds her subtle influence on all of this, adding to the variables. It's no wonder that every herbalist creates unique herbal preparations, and that non-herbalists feel confused.

After years of experimenting and teaching, I offer these easy, foolproof instructions for home preparation of herbal medicines. All the equipment you need is probably already at hand: canning jars with lids, small jars with lids or corks, a sharp knife, a grater, several pots and pans, water, oil, vodka, labels, and a ballpoint pen.

I prepare herbal medicines in three bases: water, spirit, and oil. Water-base products are teas, infusions, decoctions, syrups, baths, enemas, fomentations, eyewashes, and douches. Spirit-base products are tinctures, liniments, vinegars, and essences. Oil-base products include essential oils, infused oils, ointments, and salves.

In all bases I use no direct heat. No herbs are ever boiled or baked. This virtually eliminates burned, fried, and ruined medicines. And the finer vibrations of the plants appreciate the care.

In a water base, dried herbs produce the best potency. Spirit bases produce superior medicinals when fresh herbs are used, although dried roots and barks are often acceptable. Oil bases absolutely require fresh plant material. Don't assume that you have no access to fresh medicinal herbs. Weed Walks in city neighborhoods and along suburban sidewalks have never failed to provide an abundance of fresh medicinal plants.

Water Bases

Our bodies are based on water and so are plants. We digest in a water base. In most instances, I prefer herbal medicines in a water base. Nourishing herbs such as Comfrey, Nettles, and Raspberry leaf are at their best when prepared in water bases, for water is best able to extract and make accessible their full range of vitamins, minerals, and nutrients.

Water-based herbal medicines spoil rapidly and must be prepared at or near the actual time of use. However, you can store dried herbs for long periods, ready to use in a water base.

Water-based preparations are called teas, tissanes, infusions, decoctions, and syrups. They may be used as soaks, baths, douches, enemas, eyewashes, poultices, compresses, and fomentations. They are all made by soaking fresh or dried plant material in water (usually boiling).

Tea is the standard water-based herbal preparation; even restaurants know how to make it. At fancy ones they call it tissane.

Use one teaspoon dried herb per cup of boiling water. Add an extra spoonful for the pot. Let it steep in your cup or the pot for up to twenty minutes. Honey, lemon, and milk are medicinal additions. (Don't give infants honey.)

Volatile herbs are easily extracted into water and therefore prepared as teas. Chamomile, Pennyroyal, Shepherd's Purse, Ginger, Anise and Fennel seeds, Valerian, Catnip, and Lobelia are some volatile herbs used in this book.

Infusion is the most medicinally potent water-based herbal preparation. There are a great many definitions and recipes for preparing infusions; some herbalists use the term interchangeably with "tea."

My medicinal infusions contain a great deal of herbal matter and are steeped for a long time. The result is a liquid much thicker and darker than an herbal tea, leaving no doubt that you are dealing with a medicine, not a breakfast drink.

Prepare infusions in pint and quart canning jars. A teapot or cup is impractical for the long brewing an infusion requires and their openings allow volatile essences and vitamins to escape. Canning jars rarely break when filled with boiling water. They make it easy to measure the amount of water used in the brew. An infusion brewed in a jar is convenient to carry along to work, school or wherever, and this increases the probability that the infusion will be consumed.

And then there's the "wonder water" effect. Wonder water sounds like a new hype, but it is an interesting principle discovered by some researchers at *Organic Gardening* Magazine. They found that plants absorbed nourishment more thoroughly and easily from water that had been boiled, poured into a jar, covered tightly, and allowed to cool. They maintained that gas molecules normally held in water interfere with the plants' rapid and complete assimilation of nutrients dissolved in the water. These dissolved gases are released upon boiling. If a jar is filled with boiling water and capped tightly, the gas molecules cannot be reabsorbed into the water from the air. This is exactly how I prepare an infusion. And I suspect that people, like plants, benefit from and respond strongly to the wonder water effect.

Herbal infusions are the basis for all the other water-based preparations mentioned in this book: decoctions, syrups, soaks, compresses, etc.

Making Herbal Infusions

Roots: Use **one ounce** (a big handful of cut-up root, or half a dozen six inch pieces of whole root) of **dried root** in a **pint jar.** Fill the jar to the top with **boiling water.** Put the lid on the jar and let it sit at room temperature for **eight hours.**

Roots are the most dense and usually the most potent part of perennial and biennial plants. The medicinal virtues of roots are often found in their alkaloid content, which dissolves quite slowly into water. This is why many herbals suggest boiling roots; the rapid movement of the water molecules bouncing against the alkaloids frees them from the cells and extracts them into the water. I have found, however, that a very long period of infusion extracts all the useful alkaloids and medicinal substances from the roots, without the careful watching necessary when they are boiled.

Some roots and barks do not contain medicinal alkaloids (or have alkaloids that we wish to avoid) and these should be infused for only an hour or two. Slippery Elm bark, and Ginger, Valerian, and Licorice root are herbs used in this book which should be steeped for this shorter time.

Barks: Prepare the same as roots.

"Bark" is a misleading word, as the usual part of the tree or shrub actually used for herbal medicines is the **inner bark,** or cambium layer, which lies between the true bark and the wood. All the nourishment and life force of the tree, passing between roots and leaves, moves through this layer, making it a rich source of valuable *resins*, sugars, and astringents. The wood and the bark are dead cells and thus contain little that is medicinally useful. Cambium cell walls are tough, requiring long brewing for full extraction of medicinal virtues.

Leaves: Use **one ounce** of **dried leaves** (two handfuls of cut-up leaves or three handfuls of whole leaves) in a **quart jar.** Fill the jar to the top with **boiling water,** put the lid on and let it steep for **four hours** at room temperature.

Leaves contain the potent healer chlorophyll. Long steeping extracts all the chlorophyll, as well as the vitamins, minerals and other medicinal components of the leaves. Steeping in a closed jar keeps the water-soluble vitamins from escaping in the steam. Some leaves are tough and leathery and need to be steeped for more than four hours; Rosemary and Uva Ursi are leaves used in this book which require longer infusing, up to eight hours. Some leaves release their medicinal factors very easily in water. Catnip, Shepherd's Purse, Lobelia, and Pennyroyal are leaves used in this book that require steeping for an hour or less.

Flowers: Place **one ounce** of **dried flowers** (two big handfuls of crumbled-up flowers) in a **quart jar.** Fill the jar to the top with **boiling water,** put on the lid and infuse for **two hours.**

Flowers are the sexual expression of the plant. They are generally delicate and volatile. Chamomile is exceptionally volatile and should be infused for no more than thirty minutes. When the stalk and leaves of the plant are used along with the flowers, as with Yarrow, Red Clover, and Skullcap, infuse for four hours, as though it were the leaves alone.

Seeds: Use **one ounce** of **dried seeds, berries, hips,** or **haws** (one to three tablespoons) in a **pint jar** and fill it to the top with **boiling water.** Screw on a lid and infuse for **no more than thirty minutes.**

Seeds are the embryo of the plant. Though they are hard and dense, like roots, they are engineered to open and release their properties immediately upon contact with water, so they do not need to be infused for a long time. In fact, if seeds are brewed for too long, bitter oils and esters are leeched out into the water and a foul-tasting brew results. Rosehips and Hawthorn berries are exceptions; they may be steeped for up to four hours.

Combination Infusions: When preparing infusions containing several herbs, it is generally best to brew the components separately so that each herb infuses for the proper length of time. This is unnecessary if the combination is all roots, or all leaves, or leaves and flowers treated like leaves, etc.

If you buy herbs which are already mixed and wish to infuse them, brew for the shortest time needed by any ingredient; for instance, a mix containing Chamomile should be steeped for no more than thirty minutes. Some medicinal potency will be lost this way, but you will avoid extracting bitter esters, oils, and resins which may cause unwanted side effects.

The Wise Woman tradition focuses on the use of **simples.** A simple is a medicine made from a single herb. When combinations are used, the formula rarely exceeds three herbs. This tradition allows for maximum feedback on the effect of each herb and rapid understanding of medicinal herbs.

Dosage: Two cups, sixteen fluid ounces, of an infusion per day is the standard dose for a person weighing 125-150 pounds. Use one cup if you weigh 65-75 pounds. Half a cup for 30-40 pounds. A quarter cup (4 tablespoons) for 15-20 pounds.

☆

Summary of Infusion Data

Plant part	Amount	Jar/water	Length of Infusion
Roots/barks	one ounce	**pint**	8 hours minimum
Leaves	one ounce	**quart**	4 hours minimum
Flowers	one ounce	**quart**	2 hours maximum
Seeds/berries	one ounce	**pint**	30 minutes maximum

Herbal Decoctions and Syrups

Decoction, or simple decoction, is my term for an infusion which has been reduced to one-half of its volume by slow evaporation. A double decoction is an infusion reduced to one-fourth of its original volume. Some herbalists use "decoction" to refer to what I call an infusion; others use it to mean something closer to tea.

Decoctions keep longer than infusions if carefully stored under refrigeration. Decoctions are more potent than infusions; this makes them invaluable when dealing with children and animals. The smaller dose is more easily administered.

Decocting is an excellent way to prepare an herb with a terrible taste, such as Yellow Dock root, so it can be consumed without gagging. Adding a bit of some nice tasting brandy or liqueur to decoctions enhances the taste and the keeping qualities.

Decoctions of roots and barks are often prepared; decoctions of leaves, flowers, or seeds are rarely prepared. Since decoctions are made by evaporation, the volatile essences and water-soluble vitamins in the leaves, flowers, and seeds are lost in the process.

I always make decoctions when I have to be in the same room as the stove for the entire evaporating time. With such a low heat, decoctions rarely burn, but if you become involved in something else, there is the danger of reducing the liquid to a scorched nothing. For a pint of infusion (two cups), about an hour is needed to reduce it by half.

Making a Decoction

• Begin by straining the plant material out of the infusion and discarding it.

• Measure the liquid.

• Heat the liquid until it begins to steam; this is before it simmers and long before it boils. Stand right there and watch for the steam to start rising. When it does, turn the heat down very low.

• Steam until the liquid is reduced to half or one-quarter of what it was in the beginning. A little stainless steel pan with measuring marks on the side is of invaluable assistance in this process, but you can also judge by the mark left on the side of the pan as the liquid level falls. Or you can measure it.

• Pour the decoction into a clean or sterile bottle.

• Label with the contents, strength, and date. Example: Simple decoction of Witch Hazel bark, Dec. '84.

• Optional: Add one tablespoon of brandy or spirit per four ounces of decoction.

• Cap well.

• Cool at room temperature, then store in the refrigerator. Some decoctions may keep for as long as a year, others ferment and sour within a few months.

Dosage: A simple decoction is four times as potent as an infusion. One cup (8 ounces) of infusion is equal to one-quarter cup (2 ounces) of a simple decoction. Use up to one tablespoonful for an infant.

Double decocting increases the strength of the infusion by a factor of sixteen (four times four). So the dose equivalent of one 8 ounce cup is only one tablespoon (½ ounce). The usual infant dose is half a teaspoon of double decoction.

Making a Syrup

Add sugar or honey to any type of decoction, and you have a syrup. The extra sweetness makes some herbs more palatable, soothes the throat, and can improve keeping qualities.

How much sugar or honey should you add? The exact amount is determined by weight. A standard for syrups is an equal amount, by weight, of sugar and decoction.

One cup (8 fluid ounces) of water or decoction, weighs half a pound (8 ounces). So one cup of decoction requires half a pound of sugar.

Honey is about twice as sweet as sugar. Use a quarter of a pound (4 ounces) of honey to every cup of decoction. One level tablespoon of honey weighs about one ounce.

- Add the sweetener to the hot liquid.
- Increase the fire until the brew just comes to a boil.
- Pour the boiling hot syrup into a bottle and cap it. Sterilized bottles reduce the risk of producing unexpected herbal fermentations. But the boiling liquid kills many yeasts in the bottle.
- Optional: Add a tablespoon of brandy, vodka, etc. to further stabilize the syrup.
- Store the syrup in the refrigerator once it cools. Syrups keep for 3-6 months.

Depending on the herbs in your original infusion, you can make a cough syrup (Comfrey root and Wild Cherry bark), an iron tonic (Yellow Dock and Dandelion roots), a soothing syrup (Valerian root), or any other medicinal syrup.

Dosage: Generally, one teaspoon of syrup is a dose for a 125-150 pound person. The dose is repeated as needed, up to 8 times daily. Use a half teaspoonful for 60-75 pound children and a quarter teaspoonful for 30 pounds or smaller.

☆

Summary of Syrup Proportions

- Begin with one pint (16 ounces) of infusion.
- Reduce the liquid to half its original amount (8 ounces).
- Add an equal amount, by weight, of sugar (8 ounces or ½ pound), or half the amount, by weight, of honey (4 ounces or 4 tablespoons).

External Uses of Infusions

A **soak** consists of an infusion that has been rewarmed after the plant material has been strained out. The affected body part is then soaked in the warm infusion.

If you soak your feet in an herbal infusion, it's a **foot bath,** an excellent way to soothe and heal the entire body, and absorb herbal benefits.

A **sitz bath** is a big soak! Two or more quarts of infusion are usually needed to fill a shallow bowl or pan big enough for you to "sitz" in.

A **bath** is an enormous soak, like steeping your body in an infusion. You can prepare an herbal bath by putting the herbs directly in the tub, but my plumber made it clear to me that herbs and drains are incompatible. Some herbals say to put the herbs in a cloth and allow the bath water to run over them but I find the resulting bath too weak. If you want a strong herbal bath, try it this way: infuse two quarts of your favorite bath herb, strain, and add the liquid to your hot bath. Ahhhhh!

Enemas, douches, and **eyewashes** are herbal infusions carefully strained and inserted into the proper body cavity.

Plant material strained out of an infusion still contains healing qualities and can be used to **poultice.** Simply place the damp plant material, warmed if desired, or fresh plant material grated, chewed, or crushed, directly on the body. Poultices are preferred for first aid and infections.

Make a **compress** by putting macerated fresh or infused dried plant material into a cloth. Compressing is recommended when using hairy herbs like Comfrey leaf which irritate sensitive skin. They are less messy than poultices, and are often the choice when dealing with internal organs and growths.

For a **fomentation,** take a clean washcloth or small cotton towel, soak it in a heated infusion, ring it out, and apply. Fomentations treat breast congestion, sprains, muscle aches, and the like.

Spirit Bases

Herbs prepared in vodka, brandy, or other liquors, or vinegar, are called **tinctures.** Tinctures can be used internally or externally. Herbs prepared in rubbing alcohol are called **liniments.** Liniments are for external use only.

Tinctures

Tinctures are a popular way of using medicinal herbs. They have the following advantages over water-based preparations:
- Tinctures remain potent for many years.

• Small quantities of tinctures are effective, sometimes as little as one drop, making them more portable and potable.

• Tinctures act very rapidly, especially when administered under the tongue.

• Certain herbal alkaloids and resins are extractable only into alcohol, not water.

• A small amount of plant material produces a tincture consisting of many medicinal doses.

Nourishing factors found in herbs, such as vitamins and minerals, are extracted into tinctures, but, since only small amounts of tinctures are taken, only small amounts of these nutrients are ingested. The Wise Woman tradition focuses on the excellent nourishment available in wild foods and herbs to support the body's ability to repair and heal itself. Thus, water-based preparations are usually my first choice as herbal medicines, but I use tinctures when I travel, when I need immediate medicinal effect, or when I am dealing with rare, horrible tasting, or expensive plants.

People who refrain from using all alcohol can still take tinctures. Since alcohol-based tincture doses are small (20 drops is an average dose) and diluted in water, the taste and effect of the alcohol is virtually non-existent. Many alcoholics indicate that herbal tinctures react like medicines in their bodies, not like alcohol. To further mitigate the effect of the alcohol, let it evaporate somewhat by adding the tincture to some water and letting it sit exposed to the air for several hours.

Dosage: Tincture dosage is widely variable. Experiment with caution and consult references.

Making a Tincture From Fresh Plant Material

The best tinctures are made from fresh plants. These tinctures are so far superior to commercial tinctures made from dried plants that they almost appear to be different medicines!

Tincturing is amazingly simple:

• Identify and pick the plant parts you desire to tincture.

• Look through the plant material and discard any damaged parts.

• Do not wash any part of the plant except roots, and those only when necessary.

• Chop the plant material coarsely, except flowers and delicate plants.

• Fill a jar to the top with the chopped plant material.

• Then fill the jar to the top with 100 proof vodka, vinegar, or the spirit of your choice. (Yes, you can fill a jar to the top twice!)

• Cap the jar tightly.

- Label the jar with the name of the plant, the part of the plant used, the type of spirit used, and the date. Example: Shepherd's Purse, whole plant in flower, 100 proof vodka, 12 May 1985.
- Top up the liquid level the next day. (The plant fairies come by and take a little taste of each new tincture.)
- Allow plant and alcohol to mingle together for six weeks or more.
- *Decant* the tincture and it is ready to use.

Making a Tincture From Dried Plant Material

Most dried plants are unsuitable for tincturing, with the exception of dried roots, resins, barks, and leathery leaves such as Rosemary, Uva Ursi, and Wintergreen. Powdered herbs are never suitable for tincturing.

The procedure is similar to making a tincture from fresh plants:
- Put two ounces of dried root or bark in a pint jar.
- Add ten fluid ounces of 100 proof vodka or other spirit.
- Cap well and label (plant, part, type of spirit, date).
- Watch the alcohol level closely for the first week and top it up as necessary. (Those fairies get very thirsty.)
- Decant the tincture after six or more weeks.

Making a Vinegar Tincture

Vinegar tinctures are not very potent, don't last for as long as alcohol tinctures, and have an aggravating tendency to rust the lid onto the tincture bottle. A few medicinal herbs, such as Lobelia and Wintergreen, are commonly tinctured in vinegar. Many garden herbs, such as Tarragon, Oregano, Chives, and Rosemary, are put up in vinegar. If you make full strength tinctures with these seasoning herbs, instead of the weak brews you've probably been making, you'll be thrilled with the marinades and salad dressings you'll be able to create.

Follow the above tincture instructions for fresh and dried plants, with these changes:
- Fill your jar to the top with room temperature, not boiling, vinegar.
- Use apple cider vinegar, wine vinegar (or wine), rice vinegar, etc., but no white vinegar.
- Use cork or plastic to cap all your vinegar tinctures. A piece of waxed paper or plastic wrap between the jar and a metal lid is acceptable.
- The usual dose of a medicinal vinegar tincture is one teaspoon per hundred pounds of body weight.
- In cooking, use your vinegar tincture just as you would regular vinegar. Heavenly!

Tips for Making All Tinctures

• Choose a jar that will be filled to the top by the plant material and the alcohol; if an empty "head space" is left, some of the plant material oxidizes and spoilage is more likely.

• For extra potency, put up tinctures when the moon is dark or new; decant them when the moon is full. This helps oils, too.

• Keep your tincture in a place where you can watch the interesting changes of color, and occasionally poke your finger in to get a taste. There is no need to shake it daily or keep it in isolation or the dark. Avoid strong direct sunlight though. Occasionally tinctures will ooze; protect your furniture.

• Although the tincture is ready to use in six weeks (that's one reason why you labeled it with the date—so you know when it is ready), there is no need to decant it then. I have kept some herbs sitting in their vodka for years with no problems or decrease of potency.

• To decant the tincture, just pour off the alcohol, put it into a brown glass bottle, and cap tightly. You will notice that the plant material remaining is still wet. Put small handfuls of it in a cotton cloth and wring, hard! (This also builds good muscles in the hands.) Add this extra tincture to your bottle.

• If your tincture is made from dried roots, much of it remains in the roots after decanting, because dried plant material absorbs alcohol. There are various ways to retrieve that extra tincture. The easiest way is to put the plant material through a centrifugal juicer (minus the cutting blade) such as an Acme or Braun. If you don't have access to a juicer, you can use a salad spinner. Wringing is also possible.

• Label the bottle of decanted tincture with the same information you put on the original tincture.

• When you're ready to use the tincture, put some of the decanted tincture in a small brown glass bottle with a dropper top. Please use only glass droppers, as residues from plastic droppers will interfere with the medicinal actions of the herbs (and your continued good health). Label the dropper bottle clearly and keep it in a safe place. Buy dropper bottles at your local pharmacy or by mail. (See References and Resources.)

• It is advisable to respect the potency of herbal tinctures; although it is unlikely that ingestion of even an entire ounce bottleful could kill someone, the likelihood of unsettling effects from such a large dose is great.

Choosing Your Spirit

I prepare nearly all of my tinctures in 100 proof vodka. Other herbalist friends wouldn't think of making a tincture in anything but brandy. Pharmacists and homeopaths make their tinctures in pure grain alcohol (198 proof).

I suggest 100 proof vodka because it is readily available and fairly inexpensive, clear, and exactly half water and half alcohol. Most books which give recommendations on dosages of tinctures assume that the tincture you are using is a 50% tincture, that is, half water and half alcohol. Preparing a tincture in 100 proof vodka eliminates the need to do fancy math to determine the correct dose.

Summary of Tincture Proportions

• Tincture **one ounce fresh** plant material in approximately **one ounce** spirit for 6 weeks.

• Tincture **one ounce dried** plant material in **five ounces** spirit for 6 weeks.

Oil Bases

There are two very different types of oil-based herbal medicines. They are known as essential oils and infused oils.

Essential oils cannot be made easily at home. They are the pure plant oil, usually extracted by chemicals or hot steam. Hundreds of pounds of fresh plant material may produce only ounces of essential oil. Essential oils are readily available commercially. They are used in aroma therapy, as insect repellents, and to increase local circulation.

Essential oils are intended for *external use*. They can be fatally poisonous if taken internally in quantity. They are also highly irritating to the mucus surfaces of the body (genitals, mouth, eyes, etc.) and may cause allergic skin reactions in some people. Be certain to keep all essential oils well out of the reach of children.

Infused oils can be made at home. They are usually reserved for external uses, but could be taken internally without disastrous results. Infused oils are much less potent than essential oils and have none of the associated side effects. Infused oils can only be made from fresh plants, with the exception of some roots which can be coaxed into an oil base if baked in the oven for many hours.

Infuse herbs in any type of oil: olive, safflower, apricot, coconut, etc. The lighter, clearer oils are expensive; they produce delicate and beautiful infused oils. Olive oil is my personal choice; it rarely turns rancid, is absorbed easily into the skin, adds its own healing benefits to the preparation, and is available inexpensively.

Making Infused Oils

- Pick the plant on a dry, sunny day.
- Discard any diseased or soiled parts. **Do not wash any part of the plant.** If there is dirt on the plant, scrub it off with a stiff, dry brush.
- Chop the plant coarsely.
- Completely fill a clean, very dry jar with the chopped herb.
- Slowly pour oil into the jar, poking with a chopstick or knife to release air and make sure oil penetrates into all layers of the herb.
- Add enough oil to thoroughly cover all the plant material and fill the jar to the very rim. (As with preparing a tincture, it is really possible to fill that jar twice: once with herb and then again with the vehicle.)
- Cork the jar or screw on a lid.
- Label the jar with the name of the plant, the plant part used, the kind of oil used, and the date. Example: St. Joan's Wort, leaf and flower, olive oil, 21 June 1985.
- Keep the jar of infusing oil at normal room temperature and on a surface that will not be ruined by seeping oil.
- Decant the infused oil in six weeks. The plants can be left in the oil longer, but have a tendency to mold and spoil if not kept very cool.
- Oil held in the plant material after the decanting can be extracted. Put small handfuls into a clean kitchen towel or cotton cloth; squeeze and wring out the oil.
- Allow the decanted oil to sit for several days while the water in it (from the fresh plant material) settles to the bottom of the jar. Then carefully siphon or pour off the oil, leaving the water behind.
- Store at cool room temperature or refrigerate.

Trouble Shooting Infused Oils

Mold grows readily in infused oils. The presence of any moisture on the herb or in the jar encourages mold growth.

- If the jar is not filled to the top, mold will grow in the air space left. To save your preparation, completely remove the mold, and fill the jar to the top with fresh oil.

• If the jar was not totally dry when you filled it, mold will grow along the inside of the jar. Save your preparation by carefully pouring the oil and plant material into a dry jar. Jars dried in the oven for five minutes immediately prior to use prevent this problem.

• If the jar is put in the sun or left near a heat source, the warmth will cause condensation inside the jar, providing the moisture necessary for colonies of mold. Remove the mold and pour oil and plant material into a fresh jar to save this.

• If the plant material was wet when combined with the oil, mold will grow throughout the oil. Saving it is impossible. Start again.

Some herbs release **gas** as they infuse. You may notice bubbles moving in the oil; this is not a problem and does not indicate spoilage. Chickweed, Comfrey, and Yellow Dock are notable in their gas production when infused in oil. The gas will force some of the oil out of the jar (yes, even if tightly capped). Corked jars go pop!

Rancidity occurs when there is plenty of heat and oxygen. Infused oils in an olive oil base resist rancidity at cool room temperature for several years. In very warm climates, adding the contents of a capsule or two of vitamin E to the decanted oil helps prevent rancidity. Tincture of Myrrh or Benzoin added to ointments also checks rancidity; use about ten drops of either per ounce of oil.

Making Ointments

Ointments and salves are easily made from infused oils.

• Pour one ounce of infused oil into a very small pan.

• Grate a tablespoon of beeswax and add it to the oil. (Buy beeswax from a local beekeeper, craft supply shop, or marine supply store.)

• Place the pan on low heat; a candle flame will suffice.

• Stir constantly until the beeswax is totally melted. This rarely takes more than a minute or two.

• Pour the liquid into your ointment jar and allow it to cool and solidify.

• If the consistency is too hard, remelt and add more infused oil.

• If the consistency is too soft, remelt and add more beeswax.

Notes

References and Resources

My Favorite Herbals:

★ *Common Herbs for Natural Health*
Juliette de Bairacli Levy; 1966, Schocken Books

★ *Healing with Herbs*
Henrietta A. Diers Rau; 1968, Arco Publishing

★ *Health Through God's Pharmacy*
Maria Treben; 1982, Wilhelm Ennsthaler, Steyr (Austria)

• *A City Herbal*
Maida Silverman; 1977, Knopf

• *A Modern Herbal*
Maude Grieve; original 1931; 1971, Dover

• *Indian Herbalogy of North America*
Alma R. Hutchens; 1969, Merco

• *The Weed Herbal*
Audrey Wynne Hatfield; original 1969; 1983, Sterling

• *Use of Plants (for the past 500 years)*
Charlotte Erichsen-Brown; 1979, Breezy Creeks Press

My Favorite Guides for Field and Garden:

• *A Field Guide to Wildflowers of NE and NC North America*
Peterson & McKenny; 1968, Houghton Mifflin

• *A Field Guide to Pacific States Wildflowers*, Peterson Series
Niehaus & Ripper; 1976, Houghton Mifflin

• *Flowers*, A Golden Guide
Zim, Martin & Freund; 1950, Western Publishing

• *Weeds*, A Golden Guide
A. Martin & Jean Zallinger; 1972, Western Publishing

- *Wild Plants for Survival in South Florida*
  Julia Morton; 1962; Trendhouse and Fairchild Tropical Gardens.

- *Edible Garden Weeds of Canada*
  Nancy Turner & Adam Szczawinski; 1978, National Museum of Canada (In USA: U. of Chicago Press)

- *Park's Success with Herbs*
  Gertrude Foster & Rosemary Louden; 1980, Park Seeds

Information on the Wise Woman Tradition:

- *Daughters of Copper Woman*
  Anne Cameron; 1981, Press Gang Publishing

- *For Her Own Good; 150 Years of the Experts' Advice to Women*
  Barbara Ehrenreich and Deidre English; 1979, Anchor/Doubleday

- *Maria Sabina, Her Life and Chants*
  Alvaro Estrada; 1981, Ross-Erikson Inc.

- *Medicine Woman*
  Lynn Andrews; 1981, Harper & Row

- *Not for Innocent Ears*
  Ruby Modesto; 1980, Sweetlight, POB 307, Arcata, CA 95521

- *Old Wives' Tales: Their History, Remedies and Spells*
  Mary Chamberlain; 1981, Virago Press

- *The Woman's Encyclopedia of Myths and Secrets*
  Barbara Walker; 1983, Harper & Row

- *When God Was a Woman*
  Merlin Stone; 1976, HBJ/Harvest

- Hygieia College
  Jeannine Parvati Baker; POB 398, Monroe, Utah, 84754

Selected Mail Order Sources for Herbs:

Avena Botanicals
POB 365
Rockport, ME 04856
"Carefully wildcrafted and organically grown herbal products."

Equinox Botanicals
Rt. 1, Box 71
Rutland, OH 45775
"The combined experience of a physician, an herbalist, and a midwife."

Frontier Cooperative Herbs
Rt. 1, Box 31
Norway, Iowa 52318
A commecial supplier; some organic herbs.

Herb Pharm
Box 116, Williams, OR 97544
"The highest quality, chemical-free, herb products possible."

Iris Herbal Products
940 Austin Ave. NE
Atlanta, GA 30307
"Source of rare and unusual flower essences; books, bottles, oils."

Meadowbrook Herbs
Whispering Pines Rd.
Wyoming, RI 02898
"Organically, biodynamically grown herbs."

Mountain Spirit
5125 Landes
Port Townsend, WA 98368
"A small home business."

Ryan Drum
Waldron Island, WA 98297
"Better herbs for better medicine." Incredible kelp!

Willow Rain Herb Farm
POB 15
Grubville, MO 63041
"Organic and wild herbs, handcrafted in a thoughtful, loving way."

Wish Garden Herbs
POB 1304
Boulder, CO 80306
"Offering products mainly made at home."

Appendix I

Herbal Sources of Vitamins

VITAMIN A: Alfalfa, Watercress, Parsley, Nettles, Violet leaves, Cayenne, Paprika, Eyebright, Raspberry leaf, Grape leaves, Dandelion, Comfrey, Chicory, Elderberries, Lamb's Quarters, Nori, Yellow Dock
Depleted by: flourescent lights, mineral oil, liver "cleansing," coffee, alcohol, cortisone, chemical drugs, excessive intake of iron, lack of available protein in the body

VITAMIN B COMPLEX: Comfrey, Red Clover, Parsley
Depleted by: sulfa drugs, sleeping pills, insecticides, estrogen, sugar, alcohol

THIAMINE, VITAMIN B1: Dandelion, Alfalfa, Red Clover, Fenugreek, Grape leaves, Parsley, Raspberry leaf, Seaweeds such as Nori and Kelp, Catnip, Watercress
Depleted by: alcohol, coffee, sugar, tobacco, narcotic drugs, raw oysters

RIBOFLAVIN, VITAMIN B2: Rose hips, Parsley, Saffron, Dandelion, Dulse, Kelp, Fenugreek
Depleted by: alcohol, coffee, sugar, tobacco, narcotic drugs, raw oysters, plus restricted diets

PYRIDOXINE, VITAMIN B6: Produced by healthy intestines; found in all whole grains
Depleted by: constipation, fasting, oral contraceptives, tobacco, radiation, pregnancy, lactation, coffee, narcotic drugs, aging, heart problems, alcohol

VITAMIN B12: Alfalfa, Comfrey, Miso, Seaweeds such as Kelp and Dulse, Catnip
Depleted by: alcohol, coffee, tobacco, narcotic drugs, laxatives

NIACIN, VITAMIN B FACTOR: Burdock root and seed, Dandelion, Alfalfa, Parsley
Depleted by: sugar, antibiotics

VITAMIN C: Elderberries, Rose hips, Watercress, Pine needles, Parsley, Cayenne, Dandelion greens, Chicory, Violet leaves, Red Clover, Burdock, Coltsfoot, Paprika, Comfrey, Plantain, Nettles, Primrose, Wormwood, Alfalfa
Depleted by: antibiotics, aspirin and other pain-relievers, coffee, cortisone, sulfa drugs, smoking anything, baking soda, mental and physical stress, infections, injuries, DDT, inhalation of petroleum fumes, aging, burns, high fevers

VITAMIN D: Alfalfa, Nettles, Sunshine
Depleted by: mineral oil

VITAMIN E: Watercress, Alfalfa, Rosehips, Raspberry leaf, Dandelion, Seaweeds
Depleted by: mineral oil, oral contraceptives, sulphates

VITAMIN K: Alfalfa, Nettles, Kelp
Depleted by: frozen foods, rancid fats, radiation, x-rays, aspirin, air pollution, antibiotics, mineral oil, enemas

Herbal Sources of Minerals

CALCIUM: Alfalfa, Red Clover, Raspberry leaf, Comfrey, Nettles, Parsley, Watercress, Cleavers, Horsetail, Coltsfoot, Plantain, Chamomile, Shepherd's Purse, Borage, Chicory, Dandelion, Kelp, Dulse
Depleted by: lack of exercise, enemas, coffee, sugar, salt, alcohol, cortisone

PHOSPHORUS: Caraway seeds, Parsley, Watercress, Nettles, Chickweed, Alfalfa, Licorice, Marigold petals, Raspberry leaf, Chicory, Dandelion, Comfrey
Depleted by: sugar, mental stress, high-fat diet

POTASSIUM: Chamomile, Comfrey, Coltsfoot, Watercress, Nettles, Dandelion, Alfalfa, Yarrow, Borage, Chicory, Eyebright, Mint, Plantain, Parsley, Kelp, Dulse
Depleted by: excessive urination or perspiration, vomiting, diarrhea, enemas, coffee, sugar, salt, alcohol

MAGNESIUM: Watercress, Alfalfa, Parsley, Primrose, Mullein, Wild Lettuce, Dulse, Carrot tops, and especially Dandelion greens
Depleted by: alcohol, chemical drugs, enemas

IRON: Nettles, Dandelion, Alfalfa, Yellow Dock, Chickweed, Burdock, Kelp, Mullein, Sorrel, Parsley, Comfrey, Chicory, Watercress, Fennel
Depleted by: lack of high-quality protein, coffee, enemas, black teas

SILICON: Spinach, Horsetail, Dandelion, Nettles, Leeks, Strawberries

MANGANESE: Alfalfa, Parsley, Spinach, Watercress
Depleted by: "cleansing" the liver

FLUORINE: Watercress, Spinach, Garlic
Depleted by: excessive calcium in the body, aluminum salts in the body

COPPER: Watercress, Alfalfa, Parsley, Kale, Nettles, Spinach, Cabbage, Chickweed (exceptionally high)

SULPHUR: Nettles, Plantain, Parsley, Coltsfoot, Garlic, Watercress, Mullein, Eyebright, Shepherd's Purse, Cabbage family vegetables, Sage

IODINE: Watercress, Parsley, Sarsaparilla, Seaweeds such as Kelp and Dulse, Mushrooms, Irish Moss

ZINC: Watercress
Depleted by: alcohol, pregnancy, oral contraceptives, air pollution

Appendix II

Herbal Preparations for the Childbearing Year

• Refer to Chapter Six for further help in making herbal preparations.

• Dosages are given for an adult weighing 125-150 pounds; adjust proportionally for heavier or lighter weights.

CONTENTS

Dong Quai Tincture

1 ounce dried Dong Quai root
½ ounce dried Comfrey root
6 inch piece Licorice root
¼ ounce dried Ginseng root (optional)

Place herbs in a pint jar and fill to the top with 100 proof vodka or Yellow Chartreuse liqueur. Seal well and label with date and contents. Enjoy watching and tasting the tincture as it grows stronger and stronger over the next six weeks. Then decant by pouring off the tincture; recover tincture trapped in the herbs by putting them through a salad spinner or juicer, or by wringing them by hand. Store the finished tincture in brown glass, out of sunlight, and away from excessive heat.

Dong Quai is one of the most effective uterine tonics and hormonal regulators known. Its action is potent and it can cause stomach distress if ingested as a simple (alone). Comfrey root protects the stomach and enhances the effect of the Dong Quai on the reproductive system by soothing and nourishing the mucus surfaces of the stomach, intestines, uterus, and ovaries. Licorice also guards against digestive disruption, but its main function in this formula is to provide precursors to needed hormones, enabling the body to balance and adjust hormone production. Ginseng is yet another root renowned for its ability to enhance and stabilize hormone production through its stimulant effect on the endocrine system.

The usual dose is 5-25 drops a day, taken in a glass of water.

Emmenagogue Formulae

• The following two formulae are in general use and seem to be erratically successful. Do not increase the amount of herb in the formulae; do not exceed the recommended dose; do not take for longer than five days; do not use both formulae together. CAUTION: Blue Cohosh may raise the blood pressure.

Emmenagogue Brew

2 tablespoons dried Blue Cohosh root
3 tablespoons dried Pennyroyal leaves
2 tablespoons dried Tansy in flower

Put the Blue Cohosh into a quart of water in a pan and bring to a boil. Put the other herbs into a quart jar. When the Blue Cohosh and water boils, pour into the jar with the other herbs. Put on a tight lid and let steep for at least 30 minutes. Strain out herbs and reheat before using.

Blue Cohosh can stimulate uterine contractions, but the responsible principle is not very soluble in water, even when the root is boiled. American Pennyroyal strongly encourages the uterus to empty out and bleed. Tansy has been used by Wise Women in Europe and the Americas for centuries to facilitate menstruation and induce abortion. Together, these three emmenagogues can produce a profuse menstrual flow in sensitive women.

The usual dose is a steaming hot cupful every four hours for up to five days, or until bleeding is well under way. The effectiveness of this formula is enhanced by the addition of a tablespoonful of brewer's yeast to every cup.

Emmenagogue Combination

20 drops Blue Cohosh tincture
20 drops Black Cohosh tincture
20 drops American Pennyroyal tincture

Measure tinctures into a cup of warm water and drink slowly. Repeat every four hours for no more than five days. Continue for one full day after bleeding starts, to insure complete expulsion of all fetal material.

Blue Cohosh tincture stimulates production of oxytocin, the hormone responsible for uterine contraction. Black Cohosh tincture enhances and supplements the action of the Blue Cohosh. Pennyroyal tincture is an old favorite for "suppressed menstruation."

Threatened Miscarriage Brew

1 tablespoon dried Black Haw root bark
or Cramp Bark
3 tablespoons dried Raspberry leaves
10 drops Wild Yam root tincture
10 drops False Unicorn root tincture
60 drops Lobelia herb tincture

Put the dried herbs in a quart jar or four cup teapot and fill vessel to the top with boiling water. Steep until cool enough to drink. Add Wild Yam and False Unicorn tinctures to one cupful of tea and drink. If contractions continue for more than thirty minutes, add sixty drops of Lobelia tincture to a second cup of tea. Drink a cup of tea every three hours, adding tinctures as needed, until miscarriage no longer threatens.

Black Haw (and Cramp Bark) sedates the uterus and can stop contractions and pain; its astringent, antispasmodic and tonic actions are best extracted in water, but you may substitute a teaspoonful of the tincture in each cup of brew. Raspberry leaves are also best used in a water base, providing calcium to ease the uterine muscles and astringency to slow bleeding.

Wild Yam root contains hormonal precursors which assist the body in creating the hormones needed to hold a pregancy; it is also an antispasmodic. False Unicorn root is the herbalist's standard for dealing with threatened miscarriage; it is reported to have been successful even when hemorrhage and regular contractions have begun.

Lobelia tincture can cause profound relaxation of the uterus and the whole body if the dose is large enough. If the 60 drops recommended here does not have a relaxing effect, increase the dose; the action of Lobelia varies widely according to the preparation used and the individual using it. Burning in the throat and a mild, but exceedingly brief, nausea accompany use of Lobelia.

Increase the effectiveness of this brew by resting in bed and taking 500 IU of vitamin E every six hours.

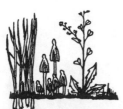

Iron Tonic

2 ounces dried Yellow Dock roots
4 tablespoons honey
2 tablespoons brandy (optional)

Put the roots into a quart jar, fill completely with boiling water, cap well. Infuse for eight hours or overnight. Strain plant material out and discard. Steam liquid over a very low flame until it is reduced to one cup. Do not boil or simmer. Add honey and stir until it dissolves. Turn up fire and bring mixture just to the boil. Pour boiling hot into a very clean jar. Add brandy or other liqueur if desired. Cap. Cool. Then store your tonic in the refrigerator.

Yellow Dock roots concentrate iron from the earth and offer it to us combined with the minerals and vitamins needed for best iron absorption in our bodies. Rises in the hematocrit (a measure of iron) of as much as a point a week are reported by women taking this iron tonic during pregnancy and after hemorrhage.

The dose is one or two tablespoons daily.

Anemia Prevention Brew

½ ounce dried Nettle leaves
½ ounce dried Parsley leaves
½ ounce dried Comfrey leaves
½ ounce dried Yellow Dock root
¼ ounce dried Peppermint leaves

Measure herbs and put them into a glass half-gallon juice jar. Pour boiling water in until the jar is totally full; cover tightly. Steep for at least eight hours.

This brew contains three excellent sources of iron: Nettle, Parsley, and Yellow Dock. It provides folic acid from the Parsley and vitamin B_{12} from the Comfrey. The green herbs all contribute vitamin C which aids iron absorption. The Mint makes it tasty.

Drink freely, up to four cups a day, for one week each month.

St. Joan's Wort Oil

Pick *Hypericum perforatum* in June, or whenever it is in full flower in your area, by cutting the top third of the plant. Klamath weed (another name) is easily recognized if you get close enough to pick a single leaf and look through it into the brightness of the sky. The clear pores and black oil glands are clearly visible and unique.

Fill any size clean, very dry jar completely full with the fresh stalks, leaves, and yellow flowers of St. Joan's Wort. Slowly add olive oil to the jar, releasing air bubbles with a knife or chopstick, until the oil reaches the rim of the jar. Cover with a good lid; label with the date. Keep at normal room temperature, out of direct sunlight, and on a shelf or other surface that won't be harmed by seeping oil. Check every week or so for mold. (See pages 138-139 for saving techniques if mold does form.)

After six weeks, pour off the reddish oil. Squeeze out oil remaining in the plant material by hand and discard the herb. Allow decanted oil to stand for several days. A thin layer of water will form on the bottom. Pour oil off the top and throw away oily water. Store the oil in a cool, dark place in a brown bottle.

Use a small amount of St. Joan's Wort oil topically for treatment of backache, stiff neck, eczema, psoriasis, sciatica, shingles, cold sores, and other skin problems. This oil is also an excellent suncreen when applied frequently.

St. Joan's Wort Tincture

Pick the flowering tops of *Hypericum perforatum* on a bright day. Pack them rather tightly into a clean glass jar. Fill the jar immediately with 100 proof vodka. Cap the jar and affix a label with the date. Watch closely and you'll see the vodka turn red! Add vodka as necessary to keep the jar absolutely full. In six weeks, pour off the dark red tincture. Discard plant material. Store well-labeled tincture in brown glass, in a cool, dark cupboard.

The usual dose is 25 drops as needed for muscle spasms. A single dose is effective in preventing muscle spasms as well as relieving them. Combined with 5 drops of Skullcap tincture, *Hypericum* tincture successfully deals with migraine and ordinary headaches, neuralgia, back pain, sciatica, temporary paralysis, and sore, stiff shoulders and neck.

Dandelion Italiano

Pick and thoroughly wash a "mess" of Dandelion (or Dandelion and Chicory) leaves. Avoid picking from roadsides, under powerlines, or in areas that have been sprayed with weed killers. Hold greens in parallel bunches and chop into half inch pieces. Put all the chopped leaves into a pan, cover them with boiling water, and then set the pan over heat until the water boils again. Drain off the water. Repeat this process once or twice more. If the greens need more cooking, add a small amount of boiling water and steam for a few minutes. Drain them well, then add several tablespoons of vinegar, a good coating of olive oil, some salt or tamari, and (optional) lots of minced Garlic or Garlic powder. Stir well, taste and correct seasoning (you'll probably need to add more vinegar). This makes a tangy, slightly bitter addition to any meal, even breakfast!

Labor Tincture

½ ounce dried Black Cohosh root
½ ounce dried Blue Cohosh root
¼ ounce dried Ginger
¼ ounce dried Birthroot
1 cup (8 fluid ounces) 100 proof vodka

Place dried herbs in a pint jar and add vodka. Label and cap. Let it all steep together for six weeks or longer. Decant the tincture by running the mixture through a juice extractor or a salad spinner. If neither of these is available, pour the tincture and herbs into a cotton cloth and wring by hand. Store decanted tincture in a cool, dark place in brown glass. Be sure to label it.

The Blue Cohosh encourages the uterus to begin contracting, and increases the force of the contractions. The Black Cohosh helps the uterus to contract in a coordinated and effective way. The Ginger focuses energy in the pelvic area, and increases the energy available to the uterus. Birthroot (*Trillium*) adds its "prompt and persistent" influence on the uterus, speeding the action of the Cohoshes and joining with the Ginger to energize the uterus.

This tincture can be used to initiate labor, strengthen contractions, unstall and stimulate labor, deal with exhaustion during labor, expel the placenta, and help control postpartum hemorrhage.

The usual dose is 10 drops under the tongue.

Postpartum Hemorrhage Formulae

• It's worth a trip to the country in May to make your own full-strength antihemorrhage tincture if you practice as a midwife. If you can't find the time or the herbs, make up a tincture from dried plants available commercially or gathered and dried for you by friends.

Antihemorrhage Tincture #1

1 part fresh Blue Cohosh roots
(or ¼ part dried roots)
1 part fresh Shepherd's Purse herb
(leaf, flowers, stalk, seeds)
1 part fresh Motherwort leaves (and stalk)
100 proof vodka or grain alcohol

In rich woods, on a bright spring day, look for the emerging "blue" leaves of Blue Cohosh. With balance and respect, gather up to a third of the slender roots. Then go to a garden or barnyard, find Shepherd's Purse in flower, even going to seed, and cut half of all the stalks you see, giving thanks. Look nearby for the maple-shaped young leaves of Motherwort. Feel and give blessing as you cut some of the square-stalked plants.

Chop the herbs coarsely and fill a jar to the top with them. Cover completely with 100 proof vodka or grain alcohol. Cap securely and label with the date and contents. This tincture is ready to decant in six weeks.

The Blue Cohosh promotes release of oxytocin and makes the uterus clamp down. The Shepherd's Purse is a fast-acting hemostatic and vasoconstrictor; it also encourages the uterus to clamp down. The Motherwort adds a calming influence to help forestall shock, and relieves pain.

The usual dose is a dropperful under the tongue, repeated in a minute if necessary.

Antihemorrhage Tincture #2

1 ounce dried Blue Cohosh roots
1 ounce dried Witch Hazel bark
½ ounce dried Valerian
   or Lady Slipper root
1½ cups (12 fluid ounces) 100 proof vodka

Place dried herbs in a pint jar, add vodka and cap tightly; label with date and contents. Let sit for six weeks or longer at room temperature. Decant by pouring off liquid, then putting wet plant material through a centrifugal juicer to thoroughly extract remaining liquid. Store in well-labeled brown glass in a cool place away from direct light.

Blue Cohosh stimulates the uterus to contract and close down rapidly. Witch Hazel is one of the most powerful and fast-acting hemostatics known. Valerian (or Lady Slipper) checks spasms and relieves pain and tension.

The usual dose is two dropperfuls, about 50 drops, under the tongue. This may be repeated in a minute if needed. And again, ten minutes later, if desired.

After-pain Brew

1 ounce dried Cramp Bark
   or Black Haw root bark
½ ounce dried Blue Cohosh root
¼ ounce dried Hops flowers

Infuse herbs in a one quart jar filled with boiling water and sealed well. After eight hours, strain out herbs and refrigerate liquid.

Cramp Bark (or Black Haw) is specific for relieving the pain of uterine contraction after birth or during the menstrual flow. Blue Cohosh helps the uterus regain its pre-pregnancy state quickly, thus reducing pain. Hops is a sleep-inducing, milk-producing pain killer.

Reheat the brew and sip it throughout the day and night, or as needed, to ease pain and encourage rest. (A little salt improves the taste.)

Postpartum Depression Brew

½ ounce dried, shredded Licorice root
1 ounce dried, crumbled Raspberry leaf
1 ounce dried, finely cut Rosemary leaves
1 ounce dried, cut Skullcap

Mix the dried herbs thoroughly together. Use two teaspoons per cup of boiling water to prepare this strongly scented and interesting tasting tea.

Licorice favorably affects the hormonal balance and cheers the spirits. Raspberry leaf tones the uterus and ovaries and increases available calcium, making life seem easier. Rosemary increases the milk flow, adds calcium, tones the liver, and is a Wise Woman favorite for depression. Skullcap is also a source of calcium and is a superb nerve strengthener and soother; prolonged use establishes emotional calm.

The usual dose is two or more cups daily for several weeks to two months.

Nursing Formula

1 ounce dried Blessed Thistle or Borage leaves
1 ounce dried Raspberry or Nettle leaves
1 teaspoon of any *one* of these seeds:
   Anise, Cumin, Fennel, Caraway, Coriander, Dill

Place leaves in a half-gallon jar and fill to the top with boiling water. Cap tightly and let steep overnight. Strain out herbs and refrigerate liquid until needed. As you get ready to nurse, pour off one cupful of the brew and heat it nearly to the boil. Pour it over a teaspoonful of any of the aromatic seeds. Let it brew and cool for five more minutes before drinking.

Blessed Thistle (or Borage) stimulates the milk flow and helps restore vitality to weary mothers. Raspberry and Nettle supply vitamins and minerals, notably calcium, needed for plentiful lactation. The aromatic seeds increase milk production and tone the digestive system; their powers are carried through the breast milk and into the child, curtailing colic and indigestion.

This brew can be drunk freely, up to two quarts a day if you desire.

Echinacea Tincture

1 ounce dried *Echinacea augustifolia* roots
or
4 ounces fresh Echinacea roots (any species)
5 fluid ounces 100 proof vodka
or spirit of your choice

Chew dried Echinacea root; if potent, it will cause a numbing, tingling sensation on the tongue.

Combine roots and vodka in a pint jar; use enough vodka to totally cover fresh roots. Seal and label. Keep at room temperature, out of direct light, for six weeks. Then pour off the tincture into a brown glass bottle. Remove what tincture remains in roots by squeezing or spinning. Label and store in a cool, dark cupboard.

I once made Echinacea tincture in a French raspberry liqueur; family and friends considered it delicious enough to be an aperitif. An Irish friend uses Jamison's whiskey. Adjust the dosage if your spirit is less than 100 proof (50% alcohol). For 80 proof tinctures, increase dosage by 10%.

The dose, preventatively, is 5-15 drops, taken two or three times a day. The dose, curatively, is up to one drop per pound of body weight, taken twice a day.

Plantain Ointment

Pick *Plantago* leaves when they are vibrant and green. Chop them coarsely and pack loosely into a clean, very dry jar. Add olive oil, dislodging air bubbles with a knife or chopstick, until the jar is filled to the very top. Label and cap securely. Let sit out of direct sunlight, on a surface that won't be marred by oozing oil.

Decant after six weeks, pouring off the oil and squeezing out what remains in the plant material. Discard the herb. Grate one tablespoon of beeswax for every ounce of oil. Stirring constantly, heat the oil and beeswax until the wax melts, usually within a minute. Pour the liquid into small, wide-mouthed jars (a good excuse for buying marinated artichoke hearts) and cool.

Use this ointment lavishly for diaper rash, insect bites, all itches, and minor wounds. It heals, stops itching, checks bleeding, and eases pain.

Glossary

alkaloid - an organic substance of alkaline properties occurring naturally in plants; generally treated by the body as a poison.

allopathic, allopathy - a healing tradition which uses chemical drugs and surgery to combat symptoms, sometimes producing iatrogenic (doctor caused) disease.

approximate - to meet nearly exactly or correctly.

astringent - an agent which contracts or shrinks body tissues, and reduces secretions and discharges.

bilirubin - a break-down by-product produced when the liver (*bili*) rids the infant of excess red (*rubin*) blood cells.

cambium - the soft tissue in the stems and roots of plants which lies between the wood and bark, and gives rise to new tissue.

carminative - an agent which expels gas from the intestines; from *carmen*, to sing.

curandera - a healing woman, a wise woman, an herbalist and spirit healer of Mexico, South America, or the southwestern USA.

decant - to pour gently from one vessel to another; to pour off and save a completed herbal tincture or oil, leaving the plant matter behind.

deva - a divine being, an angel, a plant spirit.

diuretic - an agent which increases the secretion and expulsion of urine, sometimes causing kidney stress and mineral depletion.

edema - abnormal accumulation of fluid in the connective tissue or body cavities.

electrolyte - a substance normally present in the body which dissociates into ions and thus facilitates the electrical conduction necessary for life.

endometrium - the lining of the uterus which is shed during menstruation or retained if implantation of a fertilized egg has occurred.

endorphin - a natural pain-killer produced by the body.

episiotomy - an incision through skin and muscles of the perineum. "Episiotomy is the most frequently performed obstetric operation in the West; one of the most intense and dramatic ways in which the territory of women's bodies is appropriated, the only operation performed on the body of a healthy woman without her consent." —*Sheila Kitzinger*

gamete - a mature sex cell, capable of mating with another and forming a new, unique life.

hemostatic - an agent that stops (*static*) bleeding (*hemo*).

homeopathy - a healing tradition based on the doctrine that like cures like. The potent but harmless essence or energy of plants is used as a healing agent.

kernicterus - brain damage resulting from too high a bilirubin level in the brain.

lochia - the normal discharge from the uterus and vagina following childbirth.

mucilaginous - having gummy, gelatinous, or gluey consistency.

os - an opening; the opening to the uterus through the cervix.

oxytocic (adjective), **oxytocin** (noun) - an agent which stimulates contraction of uterine muscle, and release of prostaglandin hormones, thus facilitating and stimulating childbirth; may cause miscarriage, poisoning, or death, if incorrectly used.

perineal (adjective), **perineum** (noun) - the area between the anal and vaginal openings; also known as the "taint" because 'taint one and 'taint the other.

pelvic disparity - the fully matured fetus' skull is too large to pass through the mother's pelvic outlet; an extremely dangerous situation.

purgative - an agent which vigorously empties the bowels, and may cause intense gripping pain.

root chakra - the center (*chakra*) of sexual and reproductive energy in the body, correlated with the genital region.

shock - the failure of the circulatory system to provide sufficient blood to all parts of the body.

suture - to sew together the edges of a wound.

symbiotic - advantageous association between parts, benefitting and strengthening both.

vasoconstrictor - an agent which narrows or constricts the blood vessels, thus raising blood pressure.

vasodilator - an agent which widens or dilates the blood vessels, thus lowering blood pressure.

INDEX